"A must-have for anyone caring for a loved one with dementia. The author documents her 18 year journey caring for her mother with Alzheimer's disease, sharing both her story and her wisdom. She recounts the challenges with great detail, and offers hope and inspiration to those on the journey today. This book is a guide to caring for a loved one with the disease but as important, it offers great examples of how to care for yourself.

Beautifully written, tremendously practical."

-ANDREA GALLAGHER, Certified Senior Advisor®; President, Senior Concerns; Co-Editor and Co-Author of *Live Smart After Fifty*

"In this remarkable book, Sherry Harris takes the reader on a gripping, emotional journey with a loved one who is dissembling rapidly despite all efforts of control. She has described many coping strategies forged from her own experiences. It is truly the ultimate survival guide."

-RONALD E. PELLETT, Alzheimer's caregiver

"I love this book because it provides unique and practical caregiving tips that I have never heard of anywhere else. Not only is Sherry insightful and helpful, Sherry also provides specific examples of *how* to achieve what she is recommending. This is great because so often, professionals will say to caregivers, "You should do this," but they never tell you how. Sherry tells you how in a concise and easy to read manner. I highly recommend this book."

-VIKI KIND, MA, Bioethicist; Author of *The Caregiver's Path to Compassionate Decision Making: Making Choices for Those Who Can't*

Adapting to Alzheimer's

Support for When Your Parent Becomes Your Child

Sherry Lynn Harris

Website: www.AlzCareSupport.com or www.Adapt2Alz.com

Because of the dynamic nature of the Internet, any web addresses or links contained
in this book may have changed since publication.

This book is intended as a reference volume only, not as a medical manual. The
information given here is designed to help you make informed decisions. The author
does not dispense medical advice or prescribe the use of any technique as a form of
treatment for physical, emotional, or medical problems without the advice of a
physician, either directly or indirectly. The intent of the author is to offer
information of a general nature to help you in your quest for emotional well-being.

ISBN: 978-0990417200

Dedication

This book is dedicated to all those who have
made the decision to become a caregiver:
I honor you as the heroes you are.

To my beloved husband and soul-mate:
thank you for your continual compassion,
understanding, love and support.

To my cherished son,
who shares his wisdom and helps me grow:
thank you giving me the profound joy
and honored role of being your mom.

To my siblings: thank you for the experiences
that bond us together in love and for
proving love can triumph over pain.

To my precious mother, who led by example
and taught me that love endures:
thank you for showing me the way
of honor and integrity throughout this journey
and for demonstrating how to find joy in adversity.

Table of Contents

Introduction

I have been writing this book about the Alzheimer's caregiving experience since my mother's diagnosis at age 63 until her death at age 81. Because of our bond, I have been blessed to be able to see the bright spots along the difficult path of caring for her throughout the progression of her disease. It is these highlights I'd like to bring to your attention, as recognizing them can make all the difference in one's acceptance of the role that fate has allocated to the Alzheimer's caregiver.

Yes, it is sometimes a grueling and painfully difficult task. But by paying attention to the glimmers of recognition, the little "bright spots," it can alter one's attitude towards both the acceptance and yes, even joy, which one can experience while giving themselves to this noble task.

Confucius said, "By three methods may we learn wisdom: First, by reflection, which is noblest; second, by imitation, which is easiest; and third by experience, which is the bitterest." My hope is that in reading this book you can change some potentially difficult experiences to much easier ones by using some of the examples given and by being well-informed about situations before they occur.

A portion of the proceeds of every book sold is donated to the Alzheimer's Association to help with the vital role they play in assisting both caregivers and those afflicted.

Most names have been changed to protect privacy.

Chapter 1
Suspicions of a Problem

*"Fear cannot be without hope
nor hope without fear."*
– Spinoza

In the beginning, Ollie began acting a little strange.

We overlooked everything because the alternative was too frightening to face. But we could no longer ignore her "eccentricities" the day her world came crashing down around her.

A thundering racket shattered the still air, terrifying in its deafening clamor. Roaring, tearing, shrieking noise blotted out all thought. Sound waves reverberated, shaking the entire area, as if a plane had just crash landed in the back of her second story condo.

Fearful of what she might find, Ollie timidly moved towards the source of the horrific clatter. Gingerly stepping forward, the floor seemed to be shifting, unstable, and somehow squishy. Could it be an earthquake? Lifting her right foot up, Ollie idly wondered why her sock was wet. She stood there awhile trying to puzzle out why her feet felt suddenly soggy. Another crash caught her attention and reminded her to move on. Turning the corner into the bathroom, the sight before her was complete and appalling devastation. The floor was gone, fallen along with the rest of the bathroom into the condo on the first floor below. Water sloshed everywhere, still spilling out of the wall faucets into the now empty space where the bathtub no longer stood. Leaning around the corner and stretching her fingers to the farthest they could reach, she could just barely turn the knobs to finally halt the flowing deluge. Horrified, Ollie gradually realized that she must have been running a bath and completely forgotten about it. The water must have been running for hours to soak the floor so thoroughly that it weakened enough to give way, dumping the entire contents of her bathroom, including the tub, into the floor below.

Denial is an emotion that sometimes affects us when we cannot face the truth. Ollie, my mom, knew that something wasn't right, but was feeling too afraid and alone to know what to do about it. She felt safest ignoring her symptoms and hoping they would go away. After all, she rationalized, most of the time she functioned just fine. However, this was a new situation of catastrophic proportions which neither of us could continue to ignore, and I knew it was time to move mom nearer to me so I could keep a closer watch over her.

Mom would never let us go into the back of her condo when my husband, Corey, young son, Dan, and I would visit. When we finally did gain admittance in order to organize her move, we found almost every square inch of the huge 15 by 20 foot room covered in a terrific jumble of hoarded papers and boxes piled four to five feet high. Only narrow pathways of tunnels allowed limited movement through the mess. We even found newspapers Mom had collected over the years, which she had refused to throw away, insisting that she wanted to look at them "when she got the time." One coping mechanism Mom used was that when the papers on her table got too overwhelming for her to deal with, she simply laid down a clean tablecloth over them and once they were out of sight, they were out of mind as well. Seeing all this, I now became seriously concerned about Mom's mind.

If God had given me the choice…would I rather have my mother linger in pain in old age, or have virtually no pain but instead a gradual loss of her memory…I would have chosen the latter.

I would have no idea of how difficult and heart-wrenching a journey it would be, for the two of us to traverse the time through concern, to fear, to horror, to resignation, and finally to loss. But at the same time, it was also a journey of bonding, loving, sharing and supporting one another through the experience.

"In Alzheimer's disease, brain cells degenerate and die, causing a steady decline in memory and mental function." (http://www.mayoclinic.com/health/alzheimers-disease/DS001 61) Over time, Alzheimer's disease causes a loss of abilities to remember, speak and write coherently, use judgment and problem solve. There are also changes in personality and behavior, such as anxiety, distrust, aggression and wandering. "Those with Alzheimer's live an average of eight years after their symptoms become noticeable to others," but depending on age and other health conditions, "survival can range from 4 to 20 years." (www.alz.org)

After an 18 year journey caring for my mom, I have some perspective that I'd like to share with others so they know in their darkest hour that it does get better, and that you can survive being a caregiver to your loved one afflicted with Alzheimer's disease.

My mom and I were always closer than the average mother and daughter. She demonstrated time and again an abundant, compassionate love for me, which brought us closer as the years went by.

Especially when I gave birth to my own child, my mother was so wise and understanding that she came to live part-time at our house for the first week to help me with the baby. Mom would arrive at 10pm, when I was so tired from the day that I'd fall into bed. Then, as the baby awoke in the night, she would change his diapers and bring him to me to breast feed him. When he was done, she would take him to his room and stay with him until he fell asleep so I could get some rest. And at nine in the morning, she would leave so that my husband and I could be alone with our new son during the day.

Talk about selfless service, Mom was a gem of thoughtful understanding. Through our shared experiences, our love and respect for one another grew.

So I wanted very much to help my mom, and found a spacious, 1600 square foot mobile home for her, with a lovely swimming pool and Jacuzzi on the grounds, located just five minutes from my house. Mom's mind was fairly clear at this time, but she had an idea it was going, so she insisted that I have my name, as well as hers, put on all of the escrow papers for her new property.

We then went to the geriatric medical center for testing. There are medications such as Aricept that can help delay the progression of Alzheimer's in the early to middle stages, so it is important to get an accurate diagnosis from a specialist. It's vital to have a geriatric physician's evaluation at this point, because situations like depression, stroke, thyroid disorder, vitamin deficiency, medication side effects and others can cause symptoms similar to Alzheimer's disease, such as the characteristic signs of memory loss and cognitive impairment. The doctors told us that Alzheimer's is a diagnosis of elimination – by process of purging other possibilities, they determine that it's most likely Alzheimer's disease. While an MRI (Magnetic Resonance Image) scan may indicate changes in the brain, the only positively conclusive means to identify Alzheimer's has been to perform an autopsy after death, where the characteristic shrinkage, plaques and tangles of the brain are seen. Now scientific studies are developing brain scans using Positron Emission Topography, or PET imaging, that indicate the plaques of Alzheimer's disease. (*Neurology*, July 11, 2012, based on studies at Duke University)

Alzheimer's Disease (AD) is "a type of dementia that causes problems with memory, thinking and behavior. Symptoms usually develop slowly and get worse over time, becoming severe enough to interfere with daily tasks. It currently affects over five million men and women in the United States." (www.alz.org) If no new treatments become available, the Alzheimer's Association projects the total will more than triple by 2050.

When we first went to the geriatric doctor for testing, Mom and I were both petrified. We were scared that we didn't know what was wrong, but we were also terrified to find out the diagnosis. While in the waiting room I even kept reminding her what day of the week it was, hoping she would remember it by the time we saw the doctor.

Sure enough, as part of the test process the doctor did ask my mother what day it was today, along with who was the president of the United States, did she know what state she lived in, how to draw the hands on a clock to indicate the time, and very basic things which, for the most part, she could answer. As we continued to periodically retest, however, we could definitely see a diminishing ability on her part to answer the questions. (A self-administered exam developed by Ohio State University can be found at www.sagetest.osu.edu.)

Many studies are searching for early indications of the disease. The Alzheimer's Association International Conference® 2014 announced studies indicating 1) that smell and eye tests show potential to detect Alzheimer's early and 2) a loss of the sense of smell was linked to cognitive decline; however, further study is needed.

The Alzheimer's Association says early warning signs of AD include forgetting significant dates and events, becoming confused more easily, having trouble dealing with money or numbers, difficulty judging spatial relationships (like judging distance when it is time to step on the car brakes), having difficulty making decisions, changes in mood and personality (like not wanting to be social because of worrying about no longer being able to follow the conversation and fit in) and having trouble expressing your thoughts such as struggling to find words (like calling a watch a "hand clock").

The first time I remember Mom having trouble finding the right word she said "You know that thing that's a hole in the ground." I couldn't guess what she meant so, hoping for more information, I replied "What kind of a hole?" She replied "One with water in it." "Oh, a pool?" I asked. "No, hot water." Ah, the word was Jacuzzi. When I was able to treat this kind of dilemma like a game of questions, it took the fear out of the fact that she was not able to find the word at the moment.

The responsibility of being a caregiver to your parent with AD is enormous and unrelenting, comparable to caring for a small child. Although many problems one encounters are similar, the dramatic difference is in how one envisions the future. When you explain something new to your child, you are confident they will eventually grasp the concept. There is no such assurance for the parent with AD, whose abilities to reason and comprehend shrink over time. While your child is increasing his vocabulary, your parent with AD will be losing hers. As your child grows older, you can expect that his behaviors will improve, as he learns mastery over his emotions and temper. For your parent with AD, acceptable conduct deteriorates, as they lose the ability to remember how they were taught to behave. With your child, you envision him growing into independence and joyfully fulfilling his potential. With your parent who has Alzheimer's, the future brings ever-diminishing abilities and even greater dependence upon you. The love you have for your child grows over the years, whereas the lifelong love you have shared with your parent can be eroded as their disease progresses and they are no longer capable of demonstrating that they return your love. (www.life-enhancement.com/article_template.asp?id=963)

In my mom's case, she and I were able to grow closer together, even throughout the numerous obstacles that the disease presented to us. This book provides many ideas on how to lovingly interact with your parent as you assist her through the journey of Alzheimer's. You may find she has some days when she's quite lucid and others when her thoughts seem to be mixed up. Sometimes she may fixate on an idea in her mind, and not let it go.

For example, a girlfriend of mine was keeping an eye on her neighbor, who she suspected might be developing Alzheimer's. One day, she found her wandering around the neighborhood, very distraught, looking for "the baby."

If you can put yourself in the impaired person's position and her way of thinking (what is real for her), you can invent a calming and helpful scenario. The neighbor thought she was responsible for looking after the baby (even though the "baby" she was thinking of was now 15 years old) and was worried that she had lost her.

If you were convinced this reality were true, would you accept someone telling you that there is no baby and she doesn't exist? Most likely, you'd reject this idea completely, and get quite upset. It's not a good idea to try to talk her out of it or convince her otherwise. Instead, use your imagination to picture yourself in this altered reality, and you can create responses that reassure her everything is all right, such as, "The parents came and picked up the baby, and the baby is fine."

She may have a follow-up question, such as, "Why didn't I see them take the baby?" to which you could reply, "They were in a hurry and asked me to let you know, and to thank you for taking care of the baby." This often calms the loved one's fears by reassuring her that the "baby" is not harmed in any way and that she is not irresponsible.

Sometimes talk of a baby implies that an impaired person needs an outlet for the nurturing aspect of her personality. A pet can be a wonderful companion for as long as she's able to care for it. A cat is quite a bit more self-sufficient than a dog, as it doesn't need to be walked or bathed, and is easy to feed.

A pet also provides a handy excuse when you want to introduce a caregiver into the home. While your loved one might protest vehemently that she doesn't need anyone to look after her, the concept that you both just want to be sure the pet is taken care of may be easier to accept.

By having someone come into the home on a regular basis, your loved one may be able to cope with living alone far longer. Be sure you carefully research and look into the references of anyone you hire to ensure they're honest and capable of providing excellent care. Home Care agencies (www.thehomecaredirectory.com) can offer licensed and bonded caregivers at hourly rates, or you may feel most comfortable with a person who is personally recommended to you. The in-home caregiver can prepare meals for your loved one, so you know she's getting proper nourishment, and can even dine with her to provide companionship. If you need someone to do light housekeeping or help with medication, you can arrange for that as well. The caregiver can also accompany your loved one to shop for food and other necessities.

A non-threatening way to familiarize your loved one with a new caregiver is to introduce the person as an acquaintance of yours. Take them both to lunch so they can converse and get to know each other in a comfortable neutral atmosphere. After lunch, go shopping at the supermarket so the caregiver learns what foods your parent prefers to eat. When you return to the home, the helper can assist your parent in putting away the groceries, thereby learning the layout of the kitchen.

If you're lucky, they'll get along together. You can then make another date for you and the caregiver to visit again. By the third visit, hopefully they're both comfortable enough with each other that they can manage just fine without you there as an intermediary. This frees up your time as well as gives you some peace of mind.

When we began to recognize the signs in Mom, we searched for reasons why this had hit our family. How could we be pummeled by such a devastating blow? It's hard to look at Mom and wonder if she could have reduced her risks of getting Alzheimer's. The scientific and medical communities are only in their infancy in studying and pinpointing the exact causes and ways to prevent the disease.

But certain things do stand out – that can impact the prospects of the brain getting wrapped up in the tangles and plaques of Alzheimer's.

Neurology (August 6, 2014) reported a large study confirmed that vitamin D deficiency is associated with dementia and Alzheimer's. Those tested who had a severe deficiency of vitamin D were 120% more likely to develop dementia or AD. The researchers plan to conduct clinical trials to determine if eating vitamin D-rich foods or supplements can delay or prevent the onset of Alzheimer's.

At this time, only head trauma has shown robust evidence as a risk factor. However, there's growing evidence that lifestyle factors influence brain health. Author Dr. Larry McCleary suggests that you can play a role by avoiding:

- Unhealthy "junk food" diets (replace with wholesome meals prepared with fresh ingredients and limited sugars). Emphasize wild salmon and cold water fish (high in omega-3s); blueberries, strawberries and spinach (neutralize oxygen-free radicals); eggs; avocados; nuts and seeds (high in magnesium); green tea or coffee (high in antioxidants); and spices like turmeric (used in curries), ginger, cinnamon, sage and rosemary. Avoid MSG (monosodium glutamate flavor enhancer). Buy organic from farmer's markets (to limit pesticide consumption).
- Chronic stress (Simplify.)
- Sleep deprivation (Get eight hours of sleep per night.)
- Head injury (Wear a helmet, use a seatbelt and guard against falls.)

- Smoking (Toxic compounds affect the brain.)
- Alcohol (Studies indicate one to six drinks per week is 54 percent better than abstinence, but two drinks per day results in a 22 percent greater chance of developing Alzheimer's.)
- Drugs (Including steroids, amphetamines, cocaine and ecstasy.)
  (McCleary, Larry. *The Brain Trust Program*. Penguin Book (USA) Inc., 2007. pg.46-81.)

In 2009, the Journal of the American Medical Association reported these findings after a five year study of 1,880 residents:

- Those who were physically active had a 33 percent lower risk of developing Alzheimer's than sedentary residents.
- Those whose diet was rich in fruits, vegetables, cereal and fish, but low in meat and dairy had a 40 percent lower risk of developing Alzheimer's disease. (www.alz.org/research/downloads/Research_Highlights.pdf)

A 21-year study conducted at the Albert Einstein College of Medicine in New York concluded that "Among cognitive activities, reading, playing board games, and playing musical instruments were associated with a lower risk of dementia."

  o Reading – 35% reduced risk of dementia
  o Doing crossword puzzle at least four days a week – 47% reduced risk of dementia
  o Dancing frequently – 76% reduced risk of dementia

Of the 11 types of physical exercise that were studied (including bicycling, swimming, playing golf and tennis) *"dancing was the only physical activity associated with a lower risk of dementia."* Ballroom dancing in particular was effective because of the complexity of concurrently listening to the music, reacting to your dance partner, remembering precise dance steps and improvising. According to Dr. Verghese "patients build up what is called 'cognitive reserve,' a resilience in the brain that seems to slow down or stop the disease's onset." (New England Journal of Medicine, June 19, 2003, Vol.348, p.2508-2516)

Our brain constantly rewires its neural pathways based upon their use: in simpler terms, the phrase "Use it or lose it" is applicable.

The reality for us at this moment in time was that Mom's testing showed she most likely had Alzheimer's. One thing we knew for sure – we were now on high alert and determined to help her in every way we could.

Chapter 2
Baby Steps

"Action is the antidote to despair."
- Joan Baez

If you've used your parent as a babysitter for your children, wean yourself off it *before* it becomes a problem. In spite of the benefits of bonding family members together and getting some time to yourself, this is one of the baby steps you need to take as your parent slips toward dementia.

Shortly before we realized Mom could no longer live alone, my husband and I went out on a date and left our nine year old son, Dan, with Grandma for the evening, as we'd been doing since he was born.

The next day, Dan confided to me that at one point during the evening, Grandma claimed that she didn't know who he was. It was clear I needed to explain her disease to him. After that, my son refused to visit her again, saying it was too hard for him to see her like this. Although he was young to make such a decision, Dan was mature and articulate for his age and I took his feelings into consideration. I knew it was getting harder for each and every one of us to cope with the changes in my mother.

Try to keep in mind that each of you has to deal with the changes in your loved one as best you can and in your own way. While you look after your parents out of a sense of responsibility as their child, don't demand too much from your spouse and children. If you continue to force them to visit and interact, they can become resentful not only of the situation,

15

but of you as well. Just graciously accept whatever they *are* able to give.

By taking lots of baby steps, you can help your loved one cope in many ways. First, simplify her environment as much as possible. The easier you make it, the longer she'll be able to deal with it. When she gets too much stimulation, too much complexity, too much information, it makes it harder to concentrate and accomplish everyday tasks.

For example, buy her a large address book and *print* the names and addresses in bold, easy-to-read letters and numbers. Delete information on anyone who has passed away. Buy her note cards, pre-stamp the envelopes and paste return address stickers on them to make it easier.

If your parent is no longer calling you, that's an indication it may be too difficult for him. Simplify the process, which allows him a greater sense of independence and control. We made up an 8½" x11" chart for Mom with the names and phone numbers of the people she liked to call, and placed it in a clear Plexiglas holder next to the telephone – easy to find and right where she needed it.

If your parent is familiar with using a cell phone, you can plug in the names and numbers for him, and oftentimes photos as well. If he's not, you can buy a special landline phone that has a place for small photographs on each number button. Pre-program the phone numbers into the phone so all your parent has to do is push the button with the photo of the person he wants to talk to and the phone automatically connects (www.alzstore.com/alzheimers/memory-phone.htm).

Simplify the process of getting dressed by going through your loved one's wardrobe and eliminate any clothes that don't fit, are worn out or need repair. You may want to limit or eliminate clothing that pulls on over her head, which is more difficult to put on. As her ability to use buttons decreases, you can replace them with Velcro closures. Use socks instead of pantyhose. Use bras with front closures and realize that eventually a bra isn't necessary and you can replace it with a front opening camisole.

Warning: Make sure you don't dispose of any clothing that has special significance to your loved one. For instance, she may have a favorite bathrobe that, after years of wear, looks dreadful to you. But if it's her favorite and represents a sense of comfort to her, you definitely want her to keep it. If you ignore this recommendation, you may be subjected to unrelenting questions about "Where is my favorite robe?" So be forewarned.

My friend gave a fancy dress away thinking that his aunt wouldn't have any opportunities to wear it after she moved into assisted living. After she arrived at her new home, she was extremely agitated to find the dress missing and insisted that he get it back for her. He couldn't understand why his aunt was so upset, but through considerable effort, he finally found the dress and returned it to her. Only then did she tell him that it was the dress she wanted to wear for her funeral.

My mom had gradually increased in size over the years, but had kept all of her size 10, 12, 14 and 16 outfits that she liked because she was "going to fit back into them one of these days." They were so out of date that we donated them to a university drama department that was thrilled to have the "period" fashions.

My aunt, who also developed Alzheimer's later, was a real fashion plate. She figured out a great system of coping with her fashion ensembles by hanging the matching blouse, slacks and belt all on the same hanger with a note attached stating what jewelry to wear with them. She was such a "fashionista" shehad no less than – can you believe it – a *dozen* pairs of black pants alone. So we made a day of fashion, with my aunt trying on every pair of pants and selecting her favorites. Instead of going to the mall, she went to her closet to choose each outfit to try on. Then she would come out to the living room and model it for us, oftentimes striking a dramatic pose. When we liked it we would exclaim "Dah-ling, you look absolutely Ravishing in that outfit, it's Definitely a Keeper." Or if the outfit was not good, we would mourn "Oooh, dear, that simply doesn't do a Thing for you. Get rid of it!" When we had whittled the pile of black pants down to only two pairs, it was far easier for her to get dressed - and we had fun doing it.

Once you simplify the items in the closet, simplify the jewelry box. For someone with such an attachment to fashion, we gave my aunt one dozen pairs of earrings, one in each color to match her various outfits. When she went looking for accessories, all she had to do was pick the color she wanted. If your parent isn't attached to fashion, she may be content with just one pair of gold earrings.

The kitchen can be an overwhelming area. Simplify it by eliminating all unnecessary utensils, pots, pans, etc. Your parent's days of cooking for others are limited, so dishes and silverware for six place settings, not twelve, should be adequate. Keep a quantity of sturdy paper plates on hand for those days when it's just easier to use paper than to wash dishes. Attaching labels to the front of the cupboards and drawers listing what each contains can be very helpful. Print labels (such as Glasses, Dishes, Silverware) in large, easy to read letters. When reading becomes a problem, attach photos of the dishes, silverware, etc. to the outside of the cupboards and drawers.

Almost everyone has at least one drawer in the kitchen that's a catch-all for various knives, peelers, tongs and other miscellaneous items. Remove the melon baller (trust me, she'll never miss it), along with anything else you feel she won't notice. You don't want her reaching into a cluttered drawer and getting cut on a knife because she didn't see it. You may also want to put cardboard sheaths over sharp knife blades.

Especially eliminate the numerous little containers used to store leftovers and leave only three (one each in small, medium and large). This discourages saving too many leftovers for too long, which she'll end up throwing out because she'd forgotten they were in the refrigerator. You can save some of the easily stored nesting containers with lids to use in sorting craft projects.

I liked to have simple foods on hand that Mom could easily fix herself. Fruits such as apples, grapes, pears, oranges and tangerines last a fairly long time. Arranged in a fruit bowl on the kitchen counter, your parent can readily see them when he's looking around the kitchen for something to eat. A fruit slicer, which you simply push down over an apple or pear, removes the core and slices fruit into ready-to-eat wedges.

Dried fruit, such as apricots and prunes, are also good to have on hand, as are trail mix and shelled nuts. Keep a couple of see-through plastic canisters on the kitchen counter filled with nuts, such as almonds, cashews or mixed nuts. You can buy them raw, and unsalted or dry roasted, which eliminates all or most of the salt.

Cheese is a good source of protein and your parent can easily add it to crackers for a quick meal or snack. Keep a couple of varieties, such as cheddar and jack, and a couple of different shapes and flavors of crackers on hand. Similarly, peanut butter and jelly should be staples on his shelf. Remind your parent that celery sticks filled with peanut butter make a healthy and tasty snack. Many vegetables are pre-washed and ready to eat now, such as sugar snap peas and already peeled baby carrots. Grape or baby tomatoes also require no preparation, other than rinsing.

Limit the number of knick-knacks around the house. You can do this slowly, by removing one item from a bookshelf, for example, each time you visit. Be sure to keep all of these items, so if you inadvertently remove one that he notices is gone and can't live without, you can easily replace it on your next visit. After a time you can choose to put these items into storage or sell or donate them.

If your parent has a lot of power tools that he should no longer be operating, ask to borrow them one at a time and don't return them until, or unless, he asks for them.

The mail can be overwhelming as well. Think about having all the utility and rent bills sent to you instead. Set up online bill pay or establish automatic withdrawals from your loved one's checking account on recurring costs. Then you're assured the water, electricity, gas, etc. won't be shut off because it wasn't paid. If your parent has numerous credit cards, cull them down to one. This eliminates many bills and advertisements sent by mail as well as cuts down confusion for your loved one and the chances of him losing cards or using them too often.

Once Mom couldn't find her wallet and I was worried because I wasn't sure exactly what she had in it. Make a photocopy of every item in her wallet in case she loses it. She should not keep her social security card in her wallet due to the possibility of identity theft. Put it in a safe place instead.

Every item you can eliminate helps your loved one manage better. Just remember that it's much easier for him to accept small, gradual changes (many that he may not even notice), and be sensitive to his desires on items he feels are vital to keep.

In spite of simplifying, your loved one may not be able to find something and think that someone has stolen it. This scenario happens often with the memory-impaired. She may even hide something to keep people from stealing it and then can't remember where she hid it. One day my mom was missing her hair curlers. She was very upset and insisted that her friend, Melvin, took them. Melvin was a sweet guy with frizzled, naturally curly hair. Puzzled as to why she'd think a man would want curlers, I asked why she thought Melvin was the culprit. She declared, "Just look at his curly hair!" We got her new curlers to use until we found the old ones and to this day we chuckle about it.

Gradually taking these baby steps helps our loved ones settle in and cope. With passing time, we take on new challenges, hoping to ease trying times and comfort those we love. With passing time, our other family members come to terms and learn to adapt, each in their own way.

It was only after ten long years of repressing the painful memory of that night at Grandma's that our son was finally moved to share the whole story with us. On that night while Grandma was looking after 9 year old Dan in her home, she walked into the living room, raised a pointed finger and looked him dead in the eye. "Who are you and what are you doing here?" she demanded.

Not only did she not recognize her grandson, she actually screamed at him and threw things at him to make him get out of her house. Not knowing what to do, Dan sat in a chair on the porch outside, surrounded by the dark night. After an hour or so, Grandma finally "came to" and asked him what he was doing sitting out there.

Dan was only nine at the time, and we can only imagine how profoundly upsetting the experience was to him. He gave us a glimpse by showing us this poignant poem he wrote that night:

Damn Alzheimer's

One day I went to Grandmother's house
But she wouldn't let me in.
What madness is this?
Don't you remember me, miss?
It is I, your grandson,
And I know you're not dumb.
Why do you ask who am I?
What is the cause of your lie?
This simply isn't funny anymore.
Hey, don't shut the door.
It's ME, your grandson,
What's wrong with you?
Don't you remember me,
Don't you know me?
I've known you my whole life.
Can't you recognize me?
Why don't you remember me?
What is wrong Grandma?
Can't you remember me at all?
I learned that day of Alzheimer's.

Chapter 3
Putting Affairs in Order

"Have the courage to face the truth.
Do the right thing because it is right.
These are the magic keys to living your life with integrity."
– W. Clement Stone

Mom's doctor referred us to a social worker, a professional who is dedicated to helping people function better in social situations. They are a resource for a variety of information you need, including day care centers, living accommodations, elder law attorneys, hospice providers, and other help. For example, she recommended that we make sure my name was on all of Mom's financial accounts. We had done this as standard procedure after Daddy had died, so I was surprised to learn that, while my name was on record at the bank, it wasn't on the substantial amount of funds deposited at the credit union.

Although Mom knew I was trying my best to take care of her, people generally have a lot of issues around money. My parents never let us know how much they had, and agreeing to put my name on Mom's accounts was unexpectedly traumatic for both of us. I resisted because I had never been responsible for so much money and was scared about it. Mom resisted because it meant that at some level she had to admit that she was having memory problems and it very tangibly represented giving up some of her independence. During earlier discussions, she was calm and rational and agreed that it was the appropriate step to take. But she became emotionally distraught, which caught me unprepared, when it was time to actually go inside and sign the paperwork.

It's vital that you add your name to the accounts while your parent is still of sound mind. Otherwise, somewhere down the road when he can no longer handle his money matters, you have no way of stepping in to manage them because you don't have the legal authorization. Consider, too, that if you don't take care of this while he's still competent, family members could protest that their parent didn't realize what he was doing because of the effects of Alzheimer's. Our lawyer firmly recommended that we get a letter from her doctor stating that Mom was of sound mind to make these decisions at this point in time, to ensure we wouldn't have any issues regarding this in the future.

I knew I had to get Mom's accounts in order now, as it would only get more difficult as time went by. As we sat in the parking lot of the credit union, we both cried. We knew at this moment we were facing the truth of what the future would most likely bring – at some point I would be taking care of my mom because she would no longer be capable.

She said, "I'm not ready to do this."

I patiently reminded her of all the times we had talked about this and how she knew it was something we needed to do. I reminded her that my name was already on the bank account, and I needed access to just one more place – the credit union.

I finally asked her what she was afraid of. Was she worried I would steal her money and leave her helpless? She admitted such a fleeting thought but agreed that no, she knew I would never do that. And so, having faced the worst possible outcome of what this action could produce, and feeling confident that it would never come to pass, we both felt a calm descend upon us, and we went in to sign the paperwork.

Even though I had always attended meetings with Mom's financial advisor, who invested Mom's money, he explained that there, too, we had to sign several forms to make it legal for me to have access to her funds if she couldn't manage them on her own.

I should mention that, while Mom was a wizard at making money in the real estate market, she was a near disaster at investing her funds elsewhere. Her financial advisor did very well for her until his death. When his partner took over however, he neglected to advise Mom to sell off previous investments which were rapidly declining and she lost many thousands of dollars. All combined, Mom would have been way ahead if she had simply stuffed the money under her mattress or in a no interest account at the bank.

In addition, like many with Alzheimer's, Mom squirreled money away. She hid it everywhere. When we cleaned my mother's files, we found money stuck in file folders among all the papers and in an old wallet that held lots of traveler's checks. Twice over the past dozen years, I received letters from companies saying they'd been trying to locate Mom because it was time to cash her bonds – things we had no record of.

When Mom and I visited the tax accountant together, Mom always ended up crying and saying she couldn't get the paperwork together and needed an extension. Like most compassionate men, he couldn't stand to see my mother cry. But, finally, the accountant (who had lost his own father to Alzheimer's disease) sent us a letter stating that if Mom didn't turn over the handling of the taxes to me, he would be forced to raise his price over a thousand dollars, because he just couldn't put himself through the trauma of dealing with Mom's incompetence any longer. This took the decision away from her and she was actually quite relieved that she didn't have to try to organize the taxes any longer.

No matter which child is given the responsibility of trustee for their parent, some friction among siblings is hard to avoid. I don't think anyone could have had a closer relationship than my sisters and I at this time, yet the lawyer explained to me that if we didn't disagree over the handling of money issues, we would be the first family not to experience difficulties in the history of his decades long practice.

Indeed, my two sisters and I disagreed, but I tried to allay their concerns. I assured them that I had Mom's best interests in mind as I sorted through options to give Mom the best care that we could, whether it was looking at the cost of places to live, or generally managing her funds.

As time goes by, you may feel a little overwhelmed by the number of issues you need to resolve. I found that if I let people know honestly the challenges I was facing in caring for my parent with Alzheimer's, they were quite understanding and helpful.

For example, I forgot to pay Mom's car license renewal once, and was slapped with a substantial penalty fee. When the staff of the DMV heard my story, they were very supportive, forgave the fee and even asked if they could help me in any other way. Their unanticipated concern and compassion really touched me.

I experienced repeated frustration when trying to resolve issues over my mother's accounts with businesses.

Talking to representatives by phone rarely worked. I found that writing honestly and politely, requesting what I needed while appealing to a sense of fairness, gave their staff the opportunity to offer help and compassion, and I received solid resolution to our problems. I highly recommend it.

In another difficult situation, I cancelled one credit card of Mom's, but got billed with late fees and finance charges, despite many calls to the company. In my letter, I briefly explained my mom's condition and asked for their help. I stated what I needed, and provided the account number and a copy of the written notification of my cancellation. I'm happy to report that this letter corrected the situation.

Mom also kept receiving a newspaper subscription we had cancelled. I had numerous problems with the staff continuously soliciting her to reinstate her subscription every time I cancelled. So I wrote the letter below to the president. (I didn't know his name, but it got through. If you can, get a name. You can call the company and ask, or try an Internet search.)

Dear Sir,

I have a difficult problem that has caused my mother and me considerable grief and which I feel you could easily amend. My mom has memory problems and has difficulty understanding, and oftentimes now, even speaking. We have cancelled this subscription several times, but unfortunately, someone again apparently talked her into another subscription.

I am the one who gets the phone calls in the middle of the night with my mom crying because she doesn't understand the bill and says she never asked for the newspaper. It is truly heart-rending, and so unnecessary.

Won't you please find it in your heart to do whatever is necessary to remove her from your subscription list and make sure she is not solicited again?

I try really hard to keep my mom as happy and as comfortable as possible, but I need your help on this matter. I trust that you are an individual of compassion and understanding and will make this happen for us.

Thank you so much for your prompt and thorough attention to this matter.
Gratefully yours

I received a very nice reply directly from the president who said he was looking after his own mother and could understand our situation. He assured me that he had taken care of the problem, and we never had trouble from them again.

Another necessary step is to sign important directives such as a "Durable Power of Attorney for Health Care" (also known as a Medical POA). If the patient is unable to make health care decisions for himself, this legally specifies who should do so.

In addition you need your parent to sign a Living Will, also known as an "Advance Directive." "These legal documents clearly express your wishes regarding the type and extent of medical and life-prolonging procedures you would permit in the event that disability leaves you unable to express them." This important step "helps ease the burden on your loved ones who may struggle to determine how, if at all, to intervene on your behalf." www.livingwill.com

The living will terminology may be helpful in

explaining to your parent why it is needed. In part, this is what it states:

"Death is as much a reality as birth, growth, maturity and old age. It is the one certainty of life. Let this statement stand as an expression of my wishes now that I am still of sound mind, for the time when I may no longer take part in decisions for my own future. If at any time I should have a terminal condition and my attending physician has determined that there can be no recovery from such condition, where the application of life-prolonging procedures would serve only to artificially prolong the dying process, I direct that such procedures be withheld or withdrawn, and that I be permitted to die naturally. I do not fear death itself as much as the indignities of deterioration, dependence and hopeless pain. I therefore ask that medication be mercifully administered to me and that any medical procedures be performed on me which are deemed necessary to provide me with comfort, care or to alleviate pain."

At the time this form is needed to go into effect, as your parent's caregiver and trustee, evaluate if the life-sustaining treatment would be able to accomplish the goal of returning your parent to an acceptable quality of life. For example, a situation which I encountered, discussed in greater detail in Chapter 21, was whether or not to give my mom antibiotics. In situations like these, Bioethicist Viki Kind recommends contemplating "would the antibiotics return her to a quality of life she would want to live?" *(The Caregiver's Path to Compassionate Decision Making)* If I had this concrete question to consider before the situation occurred in the later stages of Mom's disease– "would the antibiotics return her to a quality of life she would want to live?" – it would have been much clearer to me that she would not have wanted them and I would have been better able to defend that decision against others who were recommending that they be administered.

These directives can be an incredibly difficult area to discuss with your loved one, but you'll feel so much better if you ask your parents what their wishes are while they're still able to express them to you.

While a lawyer may try to convince you he needs to draw up a living will (at a substantial fee), our doctors said it was far preferable to sign a simple standard form available on various websites, such as the newer POLST form. Not every state has an approved POLST. California uses a POLST: Physician's Orders for Life Sustaining Treatment, while in New York it is called a MOLST: Medical Orders for Life-Sustaining Treatment. The POLST form is a supplement to the advance directive and it is usually signed by either the doctor or both the doctor and the patient. Check the guidelines and obtain the POLST for your State at www.polst.org. Without this form, much time can be lost because the hospital must deliberate over the interpretation of a lawyer's living will, which is usually far more complicated. And the end result may not be what you want. For instance, if the hospital connects life support systems, which is legally allowed while waiting for a determination, it can be extremely difficult to get them disconnected.

This situation was easier for me knowing what a close friend of Mom's went through. Nell suffered a stroke and the hospital put her on life support machines which kept her breathing and fed her intravenously. A few months later, when it was obvious to the doctors that Nell's condition would not improve, her daughters asked the hospital staff to remove the machines and allow her to die. Incredibly, the hospital refused. Not until the depletion of every cent of her insurance and personal funds, and the indescribable impact to her quality of life, did the hospital finally grant authorization to take Nell off life support. Her daughters were forced to endure the prolonging of their mother's life when they were left with no hope for improvement.

If you haven't prepared for this possibility by completing the proper legal documentation, you could be subjected to a similarly horrible situation. Most hospitals now have an Ethics committee which can assist you if you encounter this type of difficulty. If your parent is in a Nursing Home, contact the Ombudsman for assistance.

When you complete these medical documents (medical POA, advance directive, and POLST) be sure you place a signed, written copy in the patient's medical file and your doctor is fully aware of it. Give copies to family, friends, and all doctor's offices, as you do not know where the patient will be at their time of need. When EMT's (Emergency Medical Technicians) come to the house in answer to an emergency, they look for this information along with the patient's medication in three main places - 1) at the patient's bedside (can be taped to the wall above the bed), 2) inside the medicine cabinet (can be taped inside the medicine cabinet door), and 3) on the refrigerator door (can be held by a strong magnet) – so keep copies in these locations as well.

My mom was very specific after her friend's situation occurred, that she was not to be resuscitated, given a feeding tube or put on a ventilator to breathe. By signing the legal document and telling me exactly what her wishes were long before the situation ever arose, Mom eased the pain out of the process. It gave me a tremendous sense of peace, knowing that I would be relieved of guilt in carrying out her instructions.

Chapter 4
Tough Brakes: The Driving Issue

"Old age is no place for sissies."
– Bette Davis

For a couple of years, Mom did fine living on her own, with me stopping by several days a week to visit. She made friends at the mobile home park and enjoyed daily swims in the pool and soaks in the Jacuzzi, all of which offered her the opportunity to interact with other people. She continued to drive, and I grew increasingly concerned about her ability to do so safely. I tried repeatedly to talk to her about this but she wouldn't listen to me.

One of the toughest things you'll ever do is take the car keys away from your parent. A car represents independence – the ability to go wherever you want, whenever you want.

Even if you can put an end to your parent driving, problems remain. For example, Mom's house was near the local bus route, but how would she remember where to catch the bus? Or even that she took the bus? Once we went to the store and I noticed Mom walking out the front entrance. I asked where she was going and she said she was looking for her car in the parking lot. It would have been a long search, since we came in *my* car and *her* car was back home!

How do you know when it's time for your parent (the one who taught *you* how to drive) to stop driving? One day, Mom was driving at dusk without any headlights. It kept getting darker and she kept ignoring our suggestions to turn on the lights.   Finally, we said *"Hey*, turn on the lights, it's dangerous to drive like this."

That's when she admitted, "I don't remember how."

Now is definitely the time to take the car away, before she can't remember where the brakes are.

Just because you know your parent is no longer a safe driver, don't expect her to admit it. Mom insisted she could manage by just following what the cars around her were doing. This was her way of coping with no longer being sure what the red and green lights meant. When she ran a red light following the car in front of her, a police officer pulled both cars over and gave them tickets.

You would think you'd have some support from government agencies to pull dangerous drivers off the road, but at this time there was none. I asked the Department of Motor Vehicles to confidentially revoke her license, without letting her know I was the one who requested it. As much as we loved each other, I knew if Mom figured out I was behind her losing her license, she'd be furious with me.

After many frustrating calls to the DMV, I wrote to them documenting her inability to operate a car safely and included a statement from her doctor.

Finally, I convinced them to give her a driver's test. If she couldn't pass, they would revoke her license. This was exactly what I needed – an expert's opinion on whether or not Mom was still competent to drive.

This old classic story sums up the situation:

Two elderly women, Ollie and Min, were out driving. They could barely see over the dashboard. As Ollie cruised through a red light, Min – the woman in the passenger seat – thought to herself, "I must be losing it; I could have sworn we *just went through a red light." After a few minutes they came to another intersection and the light was red, and again Ollie drove right through. Min was convinced she was "losing it." She decided to pay very close attention to the next light. Sure enough, the light was definitely red and they went right through. Alarmed, Min said, "Ollie! Did you know we just ran three red lights in a row? You could have killed us!" Ollie turned to her and said, "Oh, am **I** driving?"*

Mom was a master at running the time out in situations she didn't want to deal with, and then calling to cry and beg for another extension on the time limit. Now her famous maneuvering and negotiating skills came into play as she missed test date after test date. She convinced the DMV to reschedule her driving test again and again, prolonging the inevitable as long as possible.

Finally, they said, "This is the last time we're rescheduling. If you miss this date, we revoke your license."

Mom, of course, didn't show up, as she could never have dealt with the humiliation of failing her driver's test. So, by default, the DMV revoked her driver's license. It was much easier for her to say she missed the test date, which kept her pride intact and retained the illusion she could drive.

In 2003, an 86-year-old driver mistook the gas pedal for the brake and sped out of control through an open-air farmer's market in Santa Monica, California. Ten people were killed and over 60 others seriously injured. (Los Angeles Times, Dec. 4, 2003)

As a result of accidents like this, many states have laws that require people to report certain medical conditions such as Alzheimer's or other dementia to the DMV. You should contact your local DMV to determine the specific laws in your particular state.

After a family conference, California physicians are required to confidentially report people who have Alzheimer's disease to the health department, (Health & Safety code section 103900) which in turn forwards the information to the DMV. The DMV determines their ability to drive by giving a visual and written test and a verbal interview. If they pass these, they move on to a driving test behind the wheel of their vehicle. www.dmv.ca.gov/about/senior/health/exercise.htm If they pass the driving test, their driver's license is generally not suspended. If they do not pass, an appeals process is available.

I'm grateful this procedure is now in place, as it takes the responsibility away from the family to report to the DMV.

Of course, just because Mom lost her license, it didn't necessarily mean she would stop driving. Old habits die hard. The DMV gave Mom an identification card to use instead of her license since you need ID for everyday living – to cash checks, get senior discounts, etc. They look quite similar and Mom insisted it *was* a driver's license. So, much to my dismay, after months of work to revoke her license, it didn't faze her at all – she kept on getting in the car and driving anyway.

Although Mom was aware that she was no longer able to do many things like she used to, as long as she had the car she still felt capable and independent. I wanted her to still have the benefit of what the car symbolized to her in the way of reassurance, but I also needed to keep her safe and off the road. My husband suggested he disconnect the distributor cap so the car wouldn't start. Who would have thought that Mom – who couldn't remember how the car's turn signals worked – could figure out how to call the auto club? After they fixed it twice, we wrote a note and taped it inside the hood saying, "WARNING: Do <u>NOT</u> fix this car. Before you do any work, you MUST call for instructions."

Surprisingly, Mom never noticed the note or, if she did, she could no longer figure out what the words meant. But a disabled car preserved her pride and dignity. It put an end to Mom's driving days with the saving grace that she decided it was all her idea. She still insisted that she could drive – she "just didn't want to right now."

While my goal is to be as kind and fair as possible to everyone involved, my primary concern as the caregiver is for my mother. The caregiver is the one close enough to understand the parent's fears of losing control of her life and her mind. Siblings who live at a distance are unable to keenly observe their parent in order to determine when they are optimistic, secure and at peace with themselves. As each instance arises, it is best to be aware when we may be projecting our own values onto the situation.

From a practical standpoint, it did make sense for someone else to be using the car. However, oftentimes the parent has a particular item which gives them a sense of security about their well-being. For a friend of mine, her mother felt it was most important to control her bathroom needs. Right up until the end, she insisted on taking care of this herself, even though it meant climbing into a wheelchair just to get to the bathroom.

For my Mom's tangled mind, her car represented that she was, at least on some level, still "okay." Many senior citizens believe that a car is taken away when the driver is considered to be a danger to themselves and others. So when I was the one given the task of explaining to Mom that one of her daughters bought the car so it could continue to be used, it was an emotionally traumatic experience for both of us. It was the only time in my entire life that I heard my mother swear using the "F" word.

After a good long cry, we tried to release the anger and frustration that Mom was not only losing her memory, but also her ability to have a say in her life and the things that directly affected her. And I had to accept that there were limits to my ability to look after her best interests.

These are the times when you have to be gentle with yourself and accept that you are doing the very best you can, and no one can expect more than that.

Chapter 5
Wanderlust

"Age is an issue of mind over matter.
If you don't mind, it doesn't matter."
– Mark Twain

Alzheimer's disease creates not only cognitive symptoms which disrupt memory, language and thinking, but also behavioral symptoms such as personality changes and agitation. (www.alz.org) This chapter addresses two issues that often occur with Alzheimer's patients and can be very disturbing to caregivers: wandering and a lack of inhibition.

Over 60 percent of people affected by dementia will experience wandering (www.alz.org). This can be impacted by the confusion they experience when they're overwhelmed by the situation they find themselves in, such as feeling lost because they don't recognize their surroundings.

If you remember ever being lost when you were a child, you probably recall the fear it engendered in you. You don't want your loved one going through that fear, so when the time comes, you won't want them exploring on their own.

The day I took my mom and young son to our local department store, Dan asked if he could go by himself to look at the toy section. I agreed, saying we would pick him up there after our shopping. Then Mom asked if she could go look at patio furniture by herself. I said I'd prefer she stay with me, not wanting to chance her getting lost. She petulantly said, "But you let your son go by himself, why can't I?"

Warning: this is where guilt overcame common sense. I said if she *promised* to stay there until I came for her, she could go. Big mistake, because once she was alone she wandered off and my son and I combed the aisles of the store until we finally found her.

The Alzheimer's Association provides a Safe Alert program where, for a fee, you can obtain an identification bracelet or necklace engraved with your loved one's name, medical conditions and a toll-free 24 hour emergency response phone number. The caregiver can call a different number (currently 1-800-625-3780) to report a missing loved one. This activates a support network, including law enforcement agencies, as well as 24-hour care counselors to help family members cope until their loved one is located. (www.alz.org)

It's also a good idea to paste a return address label in your loved one's shoes. If she's walking, she's generally wearing shoes.

My mom liked to wear pretty colored necklaces, so I got her dog tags from the local pet store and chose an assortment of pretty colors and shapes. In addition to engraving her name, address and phone number on one side, I inscribed *"Memory Impaired"* on the other.

If you are caring for your loved one at home, try placing a black mat in front of doors for wanderers. The Alzheimer-impaired mind often interprets this as a black hole, so she usually decides not to go out the door because she doesn't want to fall into the hole.

Similarly, if you place an additional door lock near the top of the door, the Alzheimer-impaired mind doesn't usually think to look there. If she tries the door and can't get it to open, even though she sees the doorknob isn't locked, she stops. She just assumes the door isn't working.

While Alzheimer's Special Care Units and many other care centers have a locked door policy to prevent your loved one from wandering off the grounds, most retirement communities don't.

If your parent is having cognitive difficulties, it's best to keep him in a familiar environment to avoid confusion. Because his brain has a limited ability to make new connections, trying to process new situations can often be overwhelming.

If your siblings live far away, you may be reluctant to put your loved one on a plane to visit them. The best alternative, of course, is to travel with them, but this may not always be possible. There are some simple steps you can take to help ensure safe travel.

While we thought Mom could still handle it, my middle sister, Genevieve, wanted Mom to come visit her at her home in Salt Lake City. Before I put Mom on the plane in Los Angeles, I made sure the flight attendants were aware of her special needs and gave her a light sedative that her physician recommended to prevent agitation.

I made Mom a necklace like a badge from a trade show, where a name card slips into a clear plastic holder. I wrote her name on the card in large printed letters. In small print, I wrote "I have memory loss." On the back I wrote my name and phone number and my sister's name, number and address.

If you use her favorite color to make the card and match the dress she's wearing to that color, she'll probably accept it as a part of her fashion ensemble. You can make it fancier by cutting the edges with scallops or adding a pretty sticker such as a flower, bird or butterfly. If your loved one is a man, get the type of badge that clips onto his shirt or suit pocket, or use an adhesive name tag.

When Mom arrived at the airport, Genevieve picked her up. Check the airline's policy. Explain your circumstances and most will arrange for an airport attendant to meet your parent with a wheelchair at the airplane door and transport her directly to you at an agreed upon location. It's appropriate, but not necessary, to give the attendant a tip – in appreciation of ensuring that your loved one wasn't left alone to wander and get lost.

Mother and daughter were happy to see each other. A couple hours into the visit Paul, an old boss of Mom's, came by my sister's house to take mom to lunch. Genevieve walked Mom out of the house and down the driveway so that Mom was ready to be picked up. She had explained Mom's situation to Paul before he arrived and made him promise to return Mom at a specific time. This would allow time for Mom to get "settled in" before Genevieve needed to leave for her first day of her new job.

Unfortunately, people who aren't familiar with Alzheimer's may not understand your concern. Particularly if your loved one is having a "good day," they may think you're overprotective and perhaps even unreasonable. Paul did *not* return Mom at the specified time, and Genevieve couldn't reach him on his cell phone.

Genevieve was in a quandary. Should she trust that when Paul brought Mom back, she could let herself into the house? Genevieve hadn't seen Mom in a long time, and Mom had seemed okay so far. She didn't want to leave for work before Mom came home, but several issues were at play here.

The opportunity for this new job came up after she had

made plans for Mom's visit, and she had worked long and hard to land it. If she didn't show up on the first day of her new job, she wouldn't have a job, and she really needed the money. If she stayed home, there was nothing she could do but wait. She decided to put a note on the door and go to work, hoping everything would be fine. All Mom had to do was walk in and make herself at home.

All parties felt their decisions were rational from their own perspectives, yet the result was a near disaster.

The former boss did return Mom to the very same place he had picked her up – the driveway in front of the house. Unfortunately, he did not see her inside. The door into the house was near the back, and nothing looked familiar to Mom. All the houses looked alike, and she didn't know where to go, so she decided to try to find Genevieve at work.

Luckily, my sister's landlord saw Mom wandering around the neighborhood. He picked her up and took her to Genevieve at work, where Mom cheerfully told my sister, "I came to help you."

Genevieve was mortified that her mommy was there, and she was put in the extremely uncomfortable position of explaining the situation to her boss and taking Mom back home.

Genevieve was scared and upset. She scolded Mom, pointing out how Mom could have gotten lost when she wandered off, and that she couldn't stay with her at work.

It was then that Mom realized the time had come to get her help, and she cried, "I need someone to take care of me." Mom's abilities to function took a turn for the worse after this ordeal, and I began to look at additional options for helping her.

Later, when my oldest sister, Stephanie, wanted Mom to join her at a resort in Colorado, I said no, based on the trauma of this last travel experience. Stephanie was extremely upset and called the doctor directly to ask him if Mom was okay to travel, to which he replied "Yes, she is." When I visited the doctor (who was new to us, as our last doctor had recently moved on), he somewhat callously asked me what my problem was – why didn't I want to send my mother to visit?

I explained that Mom didn't do well when she was taken out of her regular routine, and that she always suffered a downturn in her abilities to cope after a stressful challenge such as a trip. His answer, unbelievable as it was to me, was, "So when she comes back, you just stay around her for a few days until she recognizes you again."

When my eldest sister wanted to know why I still wasn't sending Mom when the doctor said it was okay, I repeated the doctor's coldhearted comment. When it finally sunk in, Stephanie realized my not sending Mom had nothing to do with being a punishment to my sister, depriving her of mom's company, but that it simply wasn't fair to put Mom through the trauma - or worth the adjustments both Mom and I would have to make once she came back home.

Now to address the second half of "wanderlust" ...the "lust" part. As your parent regresses in age, she may no longer remember the moral teachings with which she was raised. Like a child, she may be more interested in what feels good at the moment, and lose the sense of modesty and decorum which you may be used to expecting from her.

For example, when Mom and I were dining at a restaurant one day, I asked if she had remembered to wear her bra and slip. Much to my surprise, she immediately looked down her blouse and lifted up her skirt to check. While I was extremely embarrassed by her actions, she was totally unconcerned about them.

When someone forgets their inhibitions, they may feel free to do whatever they want, and that includes running around without their clothes on.

One friend told me how she was called to come over and pick up her father from a retirement facility because the staff said his behavior was unacceptable. When she inquired as to what he was doing, they replied that he was standing "buck naked" in the lobby and "spitting peanuts at people."

As she was driving over, she reasoned that, okay, she could understand the nudity, but she just couldn't figure out the second part of the story – why on earth would her dad be "spitting peanuts"? When she arrived and questioned the staff, they said that because of his state of nakedness, they had tried to lure him back into his room with candy M&Ms. It turned out that they used peanut M&Ms and her father didn't like peanuts: hence, he was eating the chocolate candy coating and then spitting the peanut part out!

When you place your loved one in a center with many other seniors they have a new opportunity to develop relationships and attachments. Later on, when Mom moved to a retirement center, I was thrilled that Mom found friends so quickly, but was initially taken aback by the affection she developed for a particular man. My mother had always been a one-man woman, and confided to me she had never been with any man other than my father, so this was a real shock to me.

Many times children have a hard time accepting that their parent may have a sex life. Even more complicated is when she may have had sex with a new partner, but afterwards forgot that it happened: then she became outraged when the partner subsequently made what she felt was an inappropriate action. Just because our parents may be older and forgetful doesn't mean their sexual life is dead. Try to remember your sense of humor and know that "this too, shall pass."

This Internet joke sums it up:

The old lady stood up in the senior citizen group, clutching her raised hand in a fist, and said, "I'll go to bed tonight with the first man who can guess what I'm holding in my hand."

The old guys blankly looked around at each other and finally one chirped up, "Is it an... elephant?"

The woman carefully peeked into her hand, then looked back up at the gentleman and replied, "Close enough."

Chapter 6
Retirement Living

"Hoping means seeing that
the outcome you want is possible,
and then working for it."
- Dr. Bernie Siegel

After Mom said she needed help, I took steps which could allow her to live independently a while longer in her mobile home. First, I realized she wasn't eating right. The food in her refrigerator seemed to stay there and rot, rather than being consumed. I arranged for the non-profit senior citizen program Meals On Wheels to deliver lunch to her, so she would at least get one balanced meal a day. This is a great program for seniors who are housebound, as volunteers not only deliver the meals but also talk with the seniors a short while, so they have some regular outside contact in addition to what family provides.

Unfortunately, each time the Meals On Wheels volunteer stopped by, Mom told them she didn't need or want their food. After she repeatedly cancelled the service and I repeatedly reinstated it, everyone got so fed up that we finally gave up on the program.

I tried hiring an in-home caregiver to stay with her, but Mom just couldn't understand why this lady was always at her house, and kept trying to get her to leave.

When we found a gas flame burning on the stove – Mom had walked away with no idea she had left it on – that

47

made us realize Mom's condition had reached the danger point.

I started going to the Alzheimer's support group offered by our medical provider, for help on what I should do. But the group was composed primarily of older spouses and only helped a limited amount. Later, I found a support group geared specifically to adult children caring for their parents with Alzheimer's, which was quite helpful. The social worker from our medical provider was a major help at this time. She explained to me that now was the time to move Mom into a retirement community (also commonly known as senior communities) where we could be more assured that she was eating properly and was safe.

A half dozen years had passed since our mom was diagnosed and because she was still so vibrant, my siblings and I all vehemently resisted this idea. We were also terrified at making our mom move against her wishes. Mom always had definite ideas about "right and wrong," had always been an extremely strong-willed individual, and ran the entire family as the matriarch.

Our dad was 15 years older than Mom and when they married, he made her promise to take care of him when he got old and never "put him in a home." So we were reluctant to infer to Mom that she was no longer competent to handle her own affairs and to do what she could interpret as being "put in a home." It did boost our efforts when Mom admitted she needed help, but of course she subsequently forgot that she had asked for it.

The social worker finally convinced us that this was the right step. Mom was now a danger to herself, she explained. If we continued to let her live on her own, we could be reported to the Protective Services Agency, which would make sure she was moved into a place we might not have any choice over and which would undoubtedly end up being much more unpleasant.

A cruel threat, maybe, but it was actually the impetus we needed to make the move, as the decision was no longer in our hands. We were now required to move Mom.

As the disease progresses, you need to make adaptations in living conditions to adjust for changes in your loved one's behavior. For most people, the first move is the most difficult. It symbolizes to both you and your loved one that in the fairly near future she will no longer be capable of living on her own or taking care of her own needs.

This is a huge adjustment for both of you. Expect resistance, not only from your loved one, but from your family members who will try desperately to avoid this new reality and, yes, resistance even from you. When our social worker said it was time, we *all* said, "Oh no, it can't be time yet." But she explained to us the importance of moving a loved one while she still has the ability to adjust to new surroundings. As time passes, it becomes more difficult for a person with Alzheimer's to process and retain new information.

You want your loved one to be able to find his room and navigate to the dining room on his own. He should be at a stage where he's capable of making new friends. Once he's made connections and has been accepted, the friends will understand when he forgets their name.

There is an old joke that speaks to this:

Two elderly ladies had been friends for many decades. Over the years they had shared all kinds of activities and adventures. Lately, their activities had been limited to meeting a few times a week to play cards.

49

One day they were playing cards when one looked at the other and said, "Now don't get mad at me…I know we've been friends for a long time…but I just can't think of your name! I've thought and thought, but I can't remember it. Please tell me what your name is."

Her friend glared at her. For at least three minutes she just stared and glared at her. Finally she said, "How soon do you need to know?"

The beauty of growing old is that it's a great equalizer. Every senior citizen has something that's not functioning at optimum levels anymore, whether it's parts of the body or the mind. If you're lucky, your loved one will find new friends that are accepting of his limitations.

As a first step, my sisters flew out to help locate the best quality place for Mom. At this stage, it is important for the retirement center to have activities and excursions that create opportunities to socialize with others. Most communities post a calendar of activities on a bulletin board for easy reference. The food is also an important aspect, so we reviewed the menus and asked about the availability of fresh fruits and vegetables. Many communities will offer you the chance to have a meal at their facility so you can easily evaluate the quality and quantity of the food served and also the surroundings.

The Internet is a good resource to start looking for an appropriate place for your loved one. For example, at www.SeniorLivingGuide.com, you can search by state, area and level of care. Each listing has a description, photo, services provided, and a printable brochure of the site.

While at this time my mom only needed to live in a senior community where meals were provided, if you have ample funds you may want to consider a continuing care community. This is a community that includes all levels of care as the disease progresses, from independent living, to assisted living (help with activities of daily living like bathing and dressing), and finally skilled nursing (24 hour a day care). The advantage is that your loved one has an easier time adjusting to their surroundings as the disease progresses, because all the common areas remain constant. The disadvantage is that they are expensive and sometimes even require a large endowment or "buy-in" fee in addition to a monthly fee.

We looked at numerous retirement communities, and finally found one that we liked whose accommodations were quite a bit more spacious than the rest. Mom's room was the size of two private rooms. One side could house Mom's bed and end tables. On the other side, we could set up a sitting area with her two couches facing each other, the coffee table between them, two recliners (one on the end of each couch), and three bookshelves covering the back wall to hold all of her "treasures."

We found the largest room we could because it was always important for my mom to feel she had lots of space. It was also more reasonably priced of all the facilities we checked out. We were concerned Mom's money might not last, so we made sure that if it ran out, Mom would still be able to stay there on Medi-Cal (California's Medicaid program which provides health insurance and long term care coverage for low income persons age 65 and over).

Telling Mom what was going to happen was one of the hardest things I've done in my life. Although I was terrified to even discuss the move, I took it one step at a time, feeling it would be unfair to just rip her out of her house and deposit her in new surroundings without some preparation.

We would sit on her couch together and I would say, "Now when we need to move, which furniture would you most like to have?"

She would play the game long enough for me to learn which items were most important to her, and then say, "But I won't be ready to do that for a long time yet."

The next visit I asked which statues and knick-knacks were most important, and so on, visit after visit, until I had a fairly good idea of what she wanted to keep with her. Even though Mom wouldn't admit it, through the repetition of this exercise, she had a pretty good idea this move was going to happen sooner than she preferred. I think this "conditioning" was helpful to us both, making for a gentler transition.

Anyone who has to do this for their parents will want to consider not only their parents' needs, but also their desires – what is most important to them.

Mom really enjoyed ice cream. And we didn't want to deprive her of her favorite food. We expected one of her major concerns about the new place would be, "What do I do when I want to eat ice cream?" Although it was difficult, we finally found a small refrigerator with a frozen section large enough to house two half gallons of ice cream. Sure enough, after the move, dishing up a bowl of ice cream whenever she wanted one was a great source of comfort to her.

Some facilities assign a current resident to be a "buddy" to help the new resident get her bearings, such as showing her where the hair dresser is or how to shoot pool in the recreation room. Ask if your residence provides this service, or if they could ask someone to do it. At the very least, they should assign a staff member for the first few times to accompany your loved so she can learn the way from her door to the dining room. Many retirement communities have assigned seating at mealtimes. This is actually helpful to the person with Alzheimer's, as a simple, repetitive routine is easiest for them to learn and repeat.

Bring something pretty and recognizable to hang on your parent's door so she can easily identify which room is hers. Feature her name and room number in large, *printed* letters which are easier for her to read. You may want to include a photograph of her. Many senior citizens hold a perception in mind of what they looked like when they were younger, so a wedding photo or high school graduation photo are the most likely pictures for them to recognize as being themselves. When new friends come to visit, this also serves as a point of reference they can use to start a conversation. For additional conversation points, make up a large chart that lists pertinent information, such as the main job he held, hobbies, where he grew up, favorite vacation spot, favorite food, what sports he played and so forth. Hang it in a prominent place.

At this stage, it may be helpful to give your loved one a calendar and write in the days you come to visit. I remember how I'd get frustrated when Mom would answer the door, "Oh, how I've missed you." One day after this comment, my frustration took over and I blurted out, "Mom, I've been here Monday, Tuesday, Wednesday, Thursday, and today is Friday. *When* have you had time to miss me?"

Although I can chuckle at this now, it helped us both tremendously when I wrote on the days of her calendar, "Sherry came for Lunch," "Sherry visits," "Sherry does puzzles," etc. Then when Mom was feeling down, she would look at the calendar and realize that I *had* been by to see her and that I would be coming again in a few days.

Don't expect that once your parent moves into her new surroundings that you won't have to contend with any difficulties. You'll still have to deal with many issues regarding her care. For example, in the beginning, Mom would call me up late at night and insist I come get her immediately and take her home or she would get on a bus by herself. It was a challenge to calm her down, which I did by explaining that I could come get her tomorrow, but it was too late now and I was already in bed. If she was willing to wait and spend the night, I would be there the next day. Luckily, by the next day, she had forgotten she even called.

But she did adjust, and jumped into opportunities to develop friendships. I remember going the first few times to the retirement center, worried about Mom trying to adapt, and there she was in the recreation area, waltzing with a partner among all the other couples, as everyone danced around the piano player, looking like she was having the time of her life.

One reality of having your forgetful parent living in a place with lots of other seniors is that some may not be honest and others may just pick up other people's things with no harm intended. You should take steps to protect your parent's belongings, such as labeling all of his clothing, just as you would when you send a child off to camp. One of the purposes of the move is to simplify his life, and limiting his amount of clothing makes it much easier to decide what to wear each day, as well as saves you the effort of so much labeling.

He doesn't need to keep much cash on hand, as the facility provides for most of his needs. People with Alzheimer's often like to hide money to keep it safe, and then forget where they hid it. (A word to the wise: Under the bed is *not* a good hiding place, as the money disappears.)

If your parent insists on keeping a small amount of cash with him, you can get a realistic-looking book with a space carved out inside where he can hide a small amount of cash. (www.hollowbookstore.com)   Then hide the book in plain sight on the bookcase.

What do you do about your mother's diamond wedding ring? This is not a problem if her ring finger has grown larger since her wedding day and she can't remove it. Otherwise, you can spend agonizing hours looking for where she put it when she took it off to wash her hands.

After one frantic afternoon looking for Mom's wedding ring, it was clear that we needed a solution to the problem.

I wasn't willing to deprive my mother of her most treasured possession and the symbol that linked her to her now-deceased husband. But I also would feel awful if Mom lost it. After much consideration, I went to a reputable jeweler and they replaced her diamond with a cubic zirconium that was almost the exact size and shape. When I took Mom to pick up her wedding ring, she was thrilled to have it back. Much to my surprise, she noticed the diamond was slightly different. I explained that this way she could keep wearing her wedding ring and we wouldn't have to worry about losing it. She seemed pleased with the solution.

Keep in mind that although *you* may not be ready for the move to a retirement community, your parent needs to make the change while she's still able to adapt. For my mother and me, it helped to write a letter telling her why we were making the move. We were doing it out of love and a desire to simplify her life and make living easier for her, and to focus on the benefits it would offer. You and your loved one may find comfort in doing this as well. In part, this is what my letter said:

You may feel like crying a little about the move. It's so hard sometimes to face change. This whole experience has been very hard. Believe me, Mom, I wish it were best to let you live in your mobile home.

But I love you too much to worry about an accident if you forget how to work the stove. Or have you be too hot or too cold because you don't remember how to work the thermostat. It's because I love you so much that I want the very best for you and I honestly, truly believe that your new home will become a lovely place for you to enjoy living.

So often lately you have expressed a desire to go to heaven and I think life has just been getting too hard. I want to make things better and easier for you so you'll want to stick around with me, and see your grandchildren grow up, and celebrate Christmas and birthdays and Easter and all the fun things we can still do together. I honestly think that once you get settled, you'll think it's a lovely place with a pretty view. They'll give you your own space to garden and you can swim in the community pool a block and a half away.

Everyone loves you so much. I know you'll make friends, and it's close enough for your best friend Lucille to visit you. And Fridays will still be our "Home Movie Night," so count on me coming to pick you up on Fridays to go to my house for "food and fun."

When I was growing up, there were times when you made me do things that I didn't want to do, but you knew it was for the best. You taught me well, Mom, and know that I would never want anything less than the best for you. I love you.

Ten years after I wrote this letter, I found that Mom had saved it inside the front cover of the revered family Bible. So I understood how much she treasured it, and how meaningful it was for her to have something she could reread in times of doubt or confusion, which reassured her that we would make it through this experience together.

Chapter 7
Remuneration

"Always aim at complete harmony
of thought and word and deed.
Always aim at purifying your thoughts
and everything will be well."
- Gandhi

Remuneration. Such an unlovely-sounding word. It doesn't slip off the tongue easily. Nor is it an easy decision to make, to take remuneration, if you are the caregiver for your loved one. If you keep your parent at home with you, you're entitled to be reimbursed for the additional work and incredible amount of time and effort that's involved. Like having a child, life as you know it will be forever changed when you accept this responsibility.

When I was having trouble handling all that was involved, I begged my relatives to take Mom to live near them and offered them payment from mom's funds to take care of her needs. None of them were prepared to accept the challenge. You'd think it would be worth some compensation to them to have me handle it, but on the contrary, they felt I should do it out of love.

And I have to admit, after being the trustee of my mother for many years, I do see an incredible amount of love that has come my way from the experience. I simply wouldn't be willing to trade so very many of the times I've shared with my mom.

In a way, I'm sorry my relatives missed out on all of the wonderful times. Moments of shared laughter and loving, an incredible bonding with my mom, and a trust that we were there for each other, to help each other through the rough spots and celebrate the many successes, even something as small as a thought successfully communicated.

I understood that I would be experiencing incredible stresses and mental exhaustion as my mother's caregiver that I wouldn't be going through if I was not caring for her. Studies show that the life expectancy of a caregiver looking after a family member with Alzheimer's is negatively impacted by the experience. To help you cope with the stress, you need to take the very best care of yourself that you can. If you fall apart, you are of no help to your loved one.

Getting an occasional massage to help release the pent up feelings so that I could decompress and enjoy life again was very helpful to me. You may find support, like I did, by talking with a counselor who can help guide us through the rough spots, like dealing with the grief of losing your precious loved one bit by bit. Take advantage of every free service you can find. My mom's medical insurance included some counseling sessions on how to cope and meetings with a social worker for advice on how to proceed at different stages. The Alzheimer's Association (www.alz.org) has chapters throughout the United States and offers valuable assistance free of charge. Many metropolitan areas have massage schools where you can get a massage by a student for a nominal fee.

If you are still having trouble coping after taking advantage of these services, talk with your doctor. I felt very inadequate at first when my doctor recommended I take medication to help me deal with the anxiety. But when I saw the marked changes it made in my life and how much better I was able to function, I realized that, for me, this was a big improvement in the quality of my life (and the lives of the loved ones around me).

Luckily, most caregivers have health insurance that covers the majority of the cost of any necessary prescription medication they may need.

If you choose to have your loved one live with you, research the cost of her living in a senior community or assisted living facility. Senior community living provides your loved one a room or apartment to live in and meals three times a day, along with a social structure of interaction with peers. Assisted living additionally helps with bathing, dressing and other needs as necessary. If you are providing these services at home, and it would cost "x" if you were to place her at a facility, you may consider remuneration for an amount under that cost.

For the sake of peace within the family, I suggest you compile figures from three facilities, average the prices, and then choose to do it for substantially less. For example, if it costs $3,000 per month to pay someone for these services, do it for a fraction of this – for example, one fourth. If your siblings argue that it isn't fair for you to get the money, point out that it's either that or the facility at four times the price or offer that they take on the responsibility. They will eventually come to the inevitable conclusion that it's a substantial savings over the alternative. It's best to choose a percentage of the cost, rather than a set amount, as when the services your parent needs increases, so will the cost, and when it does you need not renegotiate if your siblings have already agreed to a percentage. I chose to find a loving environment for my mom other than my home, as I knew the issue of remuneration was fraught with painful difficulties.

You might be surprised, but it's human nature, I think, to feel less anger at this being our lot in life if we're getting some compensation for all of our hard work, patience and perseverance. You'll be surprised how much it helps, when you're ready to tear your hair out with frustration, to go get a massage or a facial and just *relax* for a while. *Take the time to allow someone else to take care of YOU.* It really helps put life in perspective, and helps you look on the bright side of the situation again.

Conversely, if you don't take any remuneration, you might have more of a tendency to allow yourself to become bitter and resentful. This is of no help to either you or your loved one. How much better for her to be in an environment where you're both enjoying one another's company as much as possible. The most important thing is to decide on a way to come to grips with remuneration, and then believe in the rightness of your decision. Worrying over this problem takes too much out of you. For most people, taking some form of remuneration, however small, helps make for a better and healthier reality.

Chapter 8
Time Out (Respite)

"Have patience with all things,
but chiefly have patience with yourself."
– Saint Francis de Sales

There came a time for me, as it may one day happen to you, when you "hit the wall" and feel you cannot go on one more day. Every weekday I would get up at 6 a.m., fight traffic starting at 7 a.m., work all day long to support my family, fight traffic to get home, visit my mom and see to her needs – who always said how much she missed me, even when I was there every day – drag myself home and after my husband kissed me hello, he would ask, "What's for dinner?"

That simple question, smacking me in the face after a long day, became almost mind-numbing to me. How did I do it for so many years? I would fix a dinner every evening as my mother had taught me, with an entrée, a starch and a vegetable, and do the laundry and dry cleaning on the weekends and try to read a story to my sweet son every night before he drifted off to sleep. More and more often, I found him saying "Mom, you're missing the words. Are you falling asleep?" Lying on the bed next to him and relaxing with the story, it became hard to focus on the words and not fall asleep myself.

I realized with numbing finality that no one was going to come to my rescue …that if I did not take care of Mom, no one else would. Out-of-area relatives who can't be there may have ideas on how things ought to be done and freely tell you what you should do to provide care. But when you're not there, and not involved in the day-to-day caregiving, when you don't know the details of the situations to base an opinion on, it's impossible to know how things ought to be done. Perhaps it's human nature, but it can be disconcerting at best and debilitating if you allow it to affect you. And if your relatives don't show gratitude for all you do, take heart. It oftentimes happens this way. Issues of guilt and sibling rivalry can cause tension and wear you down. Realize that your best support may not come from your siblings, and look elsewhere to find encouragement, such as a caregiver support group, your doctor or your clergy.

As the long days wore on I became increasingly weary. I would wake up in the night, unable to sleep, worried that I had not finished my computer reports for the office or didn't have time to respond to voice messages and e-mails from my co-workers. It became harder to exist, and I often burst into tears of anger and frustration until one day while driving I knew I had to step on the brake for the red light but I contemplated not bothering, just going through the light to see if I would be killed and my burdens at last laid aside.

This is why there is such a thing called "respite care." When you are so exhausted mentally and physically that you just can't see how you can take another step or go another hour, you need to get away from it all. Nursing homes and some residential homes will take care of your loved one for a week while you get away. You may even be able to hire an in-home caregiver for a one week respite. Go by yourself, because for once you need to take care of just you and no one else. Go somewhere beautiful and peaceful and quiet and relearn what it is to sleep, fully and deeply, and awaken

64

without dread hitting you as soon as you are conscious.

Many churches sponsor retreats where the cost is on a "love offering" basis – that is, you pay what you can afford. Many hotels offer serene atmospheres where you can accomplish what you need to by simply sitting on the porch or balcony and absorbing the quiet beauty of the nature around you.

When I went on retreat, I was allowed to be by myself to sleep and heal and think and walk in nature. With no one clamoring for my attention to fulfill their needs, I was able to sleep long hours, and take naps when I wanted. I ate the food put in front of me, grateful that I didn't have to decide what to eat or how to cook it – the only energy I expended was to chew and swallow.

Instead of feeling trapped in what my world had narrowed down to, I needed to once again become aware of the world around me. To look at the sky and marvel at its hues. To walk among the wildflowers and absorb the silent strength of the mountains. To hear the joyful call of the birds and the happy gurgling sounds of the stream. To watch the snowflakes fall and twirl beneath them. To realize that all the beauty of life still exists, and I need only remember to slow down enough to take the time to see it all around me.

You'll probably need at least five days to totally unwind, let the anxiety drain out of your muscles and mind, and rebuild your inner peace. Taking your physical body to a new place, far removed from your daily routine, allows you to see differently, and gives yourself permission to just "be." Don't watch television or movies, which distract from your purpose. You can play soft, soothing instrumental music which still allows you to think as you drift with the notes. You may want to try getting a relaxing massage at the beginning, to help you let go. Try soaking in a hot tub and feel all your worries float off into the water, and let them go down the drain, emerging fresh and renewed.

This is a process of rebirth for you. A conscious act of stepping out of the person you have been and stepping into a new way of being.

Learn to breathe again. That's right, I said *breathe*. Take some time each day, and whenever you start to feel overwhelmed, just sit quietly and think of nothing but your breathing. As you breathe in, take in all of the good that's around you. Breathe in the sky, for instance. As you breathe out, relax your shoulders and your body and allow all the negativity flow out of you and float away. It's amazing how helpful this can be.

When you return home, continue to support yourself by reading uplifting stories. The *Chicken Soup for the Soul* series of books is great for this. I also like reading about heroes profiled in *Reader's Digest* magazine. *Daily Word* gives an uplifting word and affirmation, with a short inspirational writing, and is a way to begin your day in a positive, encouraging way. You can access it online at www.dailyword. com.

Try doing this yoga blessing. Outdoors is best.

I use it to start my day.

Yoga Blessing
- Stand up straight and inhale deeply, stretching your arms up to the sky and then press your palms together over your head.
- As you exhale, bend your elbows to bring your

hands down, touching your thumbs to your forehead to remind you to quiet your mind, then continue bringing your hands down to the front of your heart, in the middle of your chest.

- Cross your hands over your heart and inhale; then hum as you exhale, and bless yourself.
- Inhale, consciously opening your heart; exhale, gently lowering your hands toward your sides, about half-way to shoulder height, palms facing front, and bless the world.
- Continue the circle of bringing your arms up over your head as you inhale, beginning the cycle again. Repeat three times.

Watch the sunrise and the sunset as often as you can. It comforts on a deep level to know that it is forever dependable, always changing yet always the same. Watching waves break or ripples in a pond is soothing in the same way. Take time to nurture and care for yourself, so you'll be able to be there for the others who depend on you.

Chapter 9
Seeking Bliss and Finding JOY

"What you focus on expands, and
when you focus on the goodness in your life,
you create more of it."
– Oprah Winfrey

You can create many enjoyable times together with your parent at the different stages of Alzheimer's disease. For many years, my mother enjoyed both swimming in the pool and soaking in the hot tub. I was careful to always observe her, especially climbing in and out of our neighborhood pool while holding onto the rail, and to be sure she still remembered how to swim. For safety, I showed her how to put a "noodle" pool toy under her arms to support her weight.

A pool noodle is a flotation device shaped like a noodle, approximately five feet long and four inches in diameter and seemed to comfortably support Mom's 200 pounds as she moved through the water by kicking her feet. In the shallow end of the pool, we would stage mock swordfights with my mom, my young son Dan and me, each wielding our limp noodles at each other, laughing unrestrained. The more you can laugh, the easier everything seems to be.

Our pool provided a shower for rinsing off before and after swimming. A word of caution: Be sure you test the water's temperature. One time we thought the water was perfect, but didn't realize it continued to heat up, until Mom was shouting as she tried to escape the now-scalding temperature. For home use, you can purchase an anti-scalding device called a Temperature Activated Flow Reducer (TAFR) which automatically turns off the water if the temperature gets too hot. (www.alzstore.com)

A benefit of an outdoor pool shower is that, if it's allowed, it's very easy to wash your parent's hair there. Sometimes seniors get scared about getting in the bathtub or shower at home – oftentimes because they're afraid of falling. Since this shower was outside, there was no step to climb over. And the surface of the ground was anti-slip, making it safer.

Because swimming meant so much to my mom – she swam almost every day – it was important for Mom to have a swimming pool wherever she lived. As you can imagine the liability issues, this was somewhat difficult as most places didn't have a pool on purpose. At the retirement facility where Mom lived, residents had privileges at the swimming pool located at the local community center, within walking distance. At first, I hired someone to take my mom, but she soon made friends with people who lived with her and they would walk to the pool together so I didn't have to worry about her getting lost.

Later on, when Mom would need additional care and we would move her to a lovely residential home, she had a beautiful swimming pool there. We gave her a flotation raft which offered more support than the fun noodle. I found, however, that just as Mom had felt immense comfort knowing her (disabled) car was parked in the driveway of her mobile home, so, too, did she get comfort from just being able to see the swimming pool and knowing she could go swim if she wanted to, rather than actually doing it.

Other joys come from simple drives. If you have the

financial ability to let your loved one keep her car even though she can't drive any more, do so. She'll enjoy a leisurely drive even more if you take her in her own car. If it's autumn and the leaves are turning, she'll enjoy looking at the colors from the familiar safety and comfort of being inside her car. My mom always loved watching the cumulous clouds, so whenever puffy white clouds filled the sky I knew it would be a good day to take her on a drive.

In springtime, take your loved one on walks through gardens so she can smell the roses. We loved inhaling the sweet fragrance of the orange blossoms when the trees were in bloom.

Explore your local parks for a restful afternoon of being with your loved one. Our favorite park had a large pond where we could feed the ducks. Flocks of birds flew overhead and we spent many happy hours watching their aerial formations.

All of these pastimes are calming activities which help soothe agitation, yet require little effort on your loved one's part to participate. Oftentimes, we would drive to the beach and spend an hour watching the waves. Don't let her go in the ocean alone, as she may not remember to never turn her back to the waves. A wave knocking Mom off balance once was enough for me. After that, we only walked along the shoreline or looked out a restaurant window at the waves, and she seemed to enjoy that just as much.

Pets can bring lots of loving interaction and studies indicate that Alzheimer's patients do well in relating to them. Mom always loved it when I brought my little Maltese dog to sit on her lap and visit with her while she gently petted him. When we moved Mom to a state-of-the-art Alzheimer's facility, a couple of dogs and cats had the run of the place, and several birds perched in cages throughout the hallways. Feeding birds in your back yard is also a fun pastime you can enjoy together.

Tuning the television to animal programs is likely to be entertaining as well, as long as you avoid creatures your parent would be afraid of, such as gigantic, hairy tarantulas. You can get copies of old television programs that they enjoyed in earlier days, such as *I Love Lucy, The Andy Griffith Show* or *The Beverly Hillbillies* – comedies that will lift their spirits while reminding them of happy times. Sentimental sing-alongs are also entertaining – many ready-made sing-along DVD resources, complete with lyrics, are available by searching on the Internet. (www.alzstore.com)

Looking at picture books is another pastime we enjoyed together. Find a subject that's important and meaningful to your loved one. It might be trains or planes or flowers or birds. Remember that even when your parent is no longer able to read, picture books can still be a source of bliss.

If they loved to go camping, get books on the nature parks and campgrounds they visited, such as Ansel Adams' photographic records of Yosemite National Park.

Magazines like *National Geographic* have spectacular pictorials, and if you read the articles, you can tell them about the stories that go with the pictures. While waiting at the doctor's office, we always had fun looking at the magazine ads and commenting on the fashions and hairstyles.

One comment about doctor visits: When your parent needs a shot, remember that she can act very childlike. To avoid possible unpleasantness, take a lollypop with you and show it to her. Let her watch you unwrap it while the doctor's getting ready to give the shot, as this will divert her attention to focus on you and the treat. At the same time he starts the injection, put the lollypop on her tongue. This worked beautifully with my mom, as one moment she was aware of a pinch of the needle, but was immediately distracted by the sensation of the lollypop's cherry flavor. I love finding little triumphs like this that can turn a difficult situation into an enjoyable one for both of you.

Remember that touch is very important, and take the opportunity to hug and kiss and hold hands with your loved one, just as she did with you when you were young.

My mom loved babies, any kind of babies. Every time we saw a baby she would comment on how adorable it was, no matter how homely it may have appeared to me. I used to take offense at this, (thinking she was not-so-subtly reprimanding me for not having more babies) until I realized that she was simply expressing her love for them. She never met a baby she didn't like. So I bought Mom the charming pictorial books by photographer Anne Geddes, who poses babies in fanciful costumes, like teddy bears, sunflowers and fairies, and we loved pouring over them together.

I thought about how much of my mom's life had been centered around caring for babies. After all, Mom had three children of her own and was one of the founders of a neighborhood nursery school co-op, which was developed because the parents couldn't find a nursery school in the area which they felt was acceptable.

I wondered how I could possibly find some way that Mom could hold a baby and thereby feel needed as well as comforted. Babies don't need words to communicate. I was absolutely thrilled to find a local program called JOY: Joining Older and Younger Generations. This program provides day care for both seniors and young children, including singing, dancing, and arts and crafts. Most remarkably, the seniors and babies have an opportunity each day to interact with one another.

You can imagine our joy the first time Mom sat in the rocking chair and was given a baby, bundled up in his blanket, to hold and rock. An expression of total bliss lit up Mom's face, as they smiled and cooed at each other, each enjoying the experience tremendously. Older toddlers enjoyed sitting on seniors' laps and experiencing – many for the first time – a little of what it's like to have a grandparent. The staff all said that the generations coming together to interact was the highlight of every day, and it was as beneficial for the youngsters as it was for the seniors.

Mom was able to attend this center and enjoy the babies for a considerable time, until her condition changed and we needed to make other arrangements. For over two years, my mom had the incredibly sweet experience of holding and rocking the babies in day care.

I urge you to contact your local Jewish Community Center, who is the sponsor, to find out if they have a similar program in your town. I was pleased to find out that whatever your religious affiliation (or non-affiliation), you are welcome to participate in their program. It certainly improved the quality of life for my mom and me, as well as for all the babies who were surrounded by Mom's love and attention.

Blissful opportunities like the JOY center did not fall into my lap. It's necessary to expend some effort to find them. As more people are living longer, more day care centers for adults are becoming available. The referral of a professional geriatric care manager – one who knows the facilities and programs available in your area – is most helpful in assisting you to find the perfect spots for your loved one.

A geriatric care manager is able to assess the level of competency of your parent and make recommendations of which facilities they think will be the best match for them. They can offer comfort and support, as well as being an expert at knowing how to point you in the right direction.

My specialist for Southern California was Nancy Wexler www.nancy-wexler.com. She was both understanding and caring.

Nancy directed me to the delightful JOY center mentioned above, as well as later on to a perfect residential home, and eventually to an exceptional Alzheimer's Special Care Unit. The money expended was well worth the advice we received.

Looking online at www.caremanager.org, you can input your zip code and find a geriatric care manager in your area who has met the professional certification standards of the National Association of Professional Care Managers. The social worker at your medical facility can be an excellent source as well – ours suggested the specific retirement community we decided on for Mom.

Remember that if you want something, it's easier to find if you aggressively pursue it. Just as the *Field of Dreams* movie says, "If you build it, they will come," keep in mind that, "If you seek bliss, you will find it."

Chapter 10
Assisted Living Assistance

"The primary cause of unhappiness
is never the situation
but your thoughts about it."
– Eckhart Tolle

When your retirement community tells you it's time to move your parent on to an assisted living facility, it can oftentimes come as a shock. While on some level I realized Mom did not smell as clean as usual, people's minds can invent all kinds of reasons to deny or ignore the truth of the changed situation, as they may have difficulty coming to grips with what this change will incur. I noticed that Mom always seemed to be wearing the same outfit, but I never realized it was because she no longer took it off, but simply slept in it and was already dressed the following day when she awakened. Sometimes it takes the administrator calling you into the office to tell you that your parent is no longer capable of bathing or dressing themselves. And that it's time to move her to a facility that will assist her in this, and other, ways.

At a loss to know where to turn or what to do, I consulted Nancy, my geriatric care manager, who explained the different types of facilities and made recommendations for my mother.

I wasn't even aware of what a board and care or residential care facility was, and Nancy explained that this was a private residence, licensed by the government to care for a maximum of just six people at a time. Some people share rooms or, for an additional fee, one can get a private room. Caregivers, who live on site, provide 24 hour a day care, do the shopping, make the meals, help the residents dress, and generally look after everything. It's very homey. The seniors all sit down to dine together, just like a family, and it usually has a fenced back yard where they can safely enjoy the outdoors.

If you check out all of the care options by yourself, be sure to ask if you can "drop by" to see the facility. Those that say you have to make an appointment first should be crossed off your list. A quality care facility will welcome you at any time and is always open about how they operate. In addition, you should be able to visit your parent whenever you want once she moves in, even on the spur of the moment, if you unexpectedly find yourself with time you could use to visit.

We had a special challenge in finding the perfect place for my mom, since we wanted both a swimming pool and a place where Mom could garden. Our care manager found the perfect spot. When I went to meet the woman who ran the board and care home, I could hardly believe our good fortune. We talked for an hour under the shaded porch overlooking the sparkling clean swimming pool, surrounded by lush landscaping, including a bright pink bougainvillea in full bloom.

The owner, Mary, was originally from Eastern Europe where people are generally raised to treat their seniors with much more respect than is customary in the U.S. She was so solicitous and caring with one resident that I actually asked her if the woman was her own mother, but she was not.

This place was spotlessly clean and absolutely

gorgeous, decorated with all of the old-world type furniture my mom had grown up with as a child. They even served the residents home-cooked meals on traditional china and silverware, seated around a sturdy dining room table. As an added bonus, the owner, her husband and her adorable seven-year-old daughter lived on site, in a separate home at the back of the property. This all seemed too good to be true, exceeded all of my best hopes and visualizations, and was definitely a place where I wanted my mother to live.

I made the arrangements for a shared room, hoping that Mom would be able to adapt until a private room became available. The big day came and Mom and I had a lovely visit with Mary. We spent a happy afternoon soaking our feet in the swimming pool and admiring the beautiful plants. Mom asked me why she was there and I honestly said, "This is such a beautiful place that I felt my mom deserved to live here." We shared dinner with the other residents, and you can bet I made an effort to learn everyone's name and be sure that they learned my mom's.

It all went well until it was time for me to go and leave Mom behind. Such a ruckus arose! Because moving to a different location involves many new situations which a brain affected by Alzheimer's has limited capability of dealing with, it usually results in a high level of anxiety. The absolute best advice I'd been given was to get a prescription from Mom's doctor for a sedative so we would have it on hand in case we needed it. Boy, did we need it! I couldn't believe this was my own sweet mother carrying on about how she wanted to go "home" – back to the retirement facility that she had so hated and complained about when she first moved in.

Luckily, my care manager had said that if we had any

problems with Mom adjusting we could call her and she would come over to assist in the transition. Nancy was a true professional, and I felt Mom was in excellent hands when I finally departed, as Mom seemed to be handling the situation much better and I was frankly totally worn out by then.

My mother was very restless in the subsequent nights at the board and care home, pacing back and forth across the room, and it disturbed her roommate. Mary, the owner, contacted the adult children of a woman with a private room to ask if they'd like to save money by moving their mother into a shared room and, luckily for us, they did. My mom was quickly transferred into her private room, where she flourished.

I think there were several reasons Mom adapted well to her new living space. It was much smaller than her previous residence, where they cared for 100 residents as opposed to just six. It was a home setting, which was more familiar to Mom. She could see the swimming pool every day, so she knew it was always available if she wanted to use it. She spent time every day absorbing the beauty of the garden, knowing that if she wanted to pull weeds or plant a flower, she was allowed to do that. Because Mom was functioning at a good level, other than needing help with bathing and dressing, Mary took her every weekday to pick up her young daughter from school. So Mom had a regular routine she could rely on and become comfortable with, which included the gentle variety of rides in the car and socialization with a child as well as adults.

Mom and I were both happy and everything went smoothly for a very long time.

Chapter 11
Choosing Your Reality

"If you change the way you look at things,
the things you look at change."
– Wayne Dyer

What can you do to lighten your load? How can you cope with the demands being put upon you? One of the biggest steps is to realize that you are not a victim in this situation. So often we allow ourselves to feel that caring for our parent was "dumped" on us...that it isn't "fair"...why should *we* be the one stuck with all of the responsibility... and so on.

My sisters said that when Mom was no longer able to live alone and we needed to move her to a care facility, that they would then take over her care from me. I remember how much I counted on this during the most difficult times, and it helped tremendously to know that there would be relief for me later on.

At the time they made the commitment, even they themselves believed it would come to pass, but it seemed far in the future...a "someday" promise. Everyone has a full life, and everyone has their own set of problems.

There is the story that God gathered people together and asked them to put all of their problems into a circle. Each person was then asked to take out whichever problems they wanted. In the end, everyone chose to take back their own set of problems.

In the movie *Hanging Up* with Meg Ryan, she takes care of her father with Alzheimer's. Meg has a great speech where she says she didn't choose to take care of her dad, but once it's thrust upon you, you learn to accept it and then to grow into it. When you reconcile yourself to the fact that you are the one, that this is your new life, you strive to make the best of it.

When I realized the burden of Mom's care was going to remain with me, I spent some time contemplating how I felt about it. In the end, I decided that I would make a conscious *choice* to take care of my mother. I realized that the bond we had forged together would take us through the challenges ahead.

This empowering song written by Daniel Nahmod (www.danielnahmod.com) was a great help to me in deciding to forgive my siblings for not taking over the care of my mother, and also in helping me to choose a life of caring for my mom.

Love Is My Decision

Love is my decision.
It's up to me to give of my heart.
Love is my decision.
No one else can tell me to start.

Love is my decision.
It's up to me to stand on that bridge.
Love is my decision.
No one else can make me forgive.

Love is my decision.
It's up to me to dance down the road.
Love is my decision.
No one else can lighten my load.

And once I decide to change my mind,
God will show me how.
Love is my decision.
My decision – right here and now.

Each individual has the ability to choose their own reality. "WHAT?" you may ask? Eastern philosophy states *it is not what happens to you that matters; instead, it is how you react to it that's important.* Do you want to view caring for your parent as a burden weighing you down? Or can you instead, shift your focus; to look at this as an opportunity to help repay your parent for giving you life, for caring and nurturing you through all of the years when you were but a helpless child. Life has come full circle, and your parent needs *your* care now.

An Internet story asks how you would feel about taking care of a little person who needed to be fed and have their diapers changed, couldn't talk, couldn't walk, and was totally dependent upon you. Then they said it is not your baby they are referring to, but rather your parent. What a difference that seems to make in the way we look at it.

If you didn't have a good relationship with your parent while you were growing up, here's your chance to do it the way you think it should be done. You have been given another chance to develop a loving relationship, as your parent depends more on you and your ability to nurture and care for them.

Choose to see the world through a loving lens, to discover beauty in hidden places, and to express a cheerful attitude and grateful heart. Is it a challenge? Absolutely. All of life is a challenge. Do things that will support you. Try singing. "Who me?" you ask. Yes. Put on some old songs you used to listen to as a teenager, and you'll remember the words like you heard them yesterday. If you are hesitant to sing, do it in the shower when no one is home. It's amazing how it can lift your spirits.

Choose some form of exercise that you enjoy and do it often. Studies have shown that as you exercise, chemicals called endorphins are released into your bloodstream, causing you to feel more content. The easiest exercise is walking, as it doesn't take any special equipment (although you might want to wear comfortable walking shoes). Instead of searching for the closest parking spot each time you go to the grocery store or mall, park farther away, and you'll automatically start getting more exercise without even making an effort to put aside a special time for it.

Try buying an exercise DVD and working out with it first thing in the morning, before you get distracted. It's an energizing way to start the day. When you get frustrated during the day, physical exercise is a healthy way to help release anger. Try buying a jump rope at the dollar store. You'll be amazed at how much harder it is to jump rope now than when you were a kid. I inherited my mother's small, portable exercise trampoline, and it does wonders to just run into the back room and jump away my frustration. Three minutes jumping on a trampoline can really make a difference in the way you feel. Think up other handy ideas that you can incorporate into your daily life.

Endorphins are also released when you eat dark chocolate. Caregiving.com states "A 2009 Swiss study found that eating 1.4 ounces of dark chocolate (about a two-inch square) every day for two weeks lowered stress hormone levels in people who were feeling highly anxious. (They ate half the dark chocolate at mid-morning and half at mid-afternoon.)

Dark chocolate also contains antioxidants (which help fight the biological effects of stress) and provides a small hit of energizing caffeine." Just don't overdo it.

Planting flowers is a nice way to give yourself a break. Tending the garden is relatively easy to do without investing much thought. It gives your mind a chance to calm down and reflect. It can be satisfying to see order in a weeded garden; to water and watch the growth of new life as the flowers bloom.

If you own a dog, walk him. It gives you time to relax mentally and physically, to unwind and notice the beauty of your surroundings. Search your local neighborhood for the most attractive places to walk. You may find a park just a few blocks away that offers a wonderful retreat from your worries. In just fifteen minutes, you can improve your state of mind, and having the unconditional love of a pet can lift your spirits.

In *Peace Is Every Step*, Buddhist teacher Thich Nhat Hanh writes "A tiny bud of a smile on your lips nourishes awareness and calms us miraculously. It returns us to the peace we thought we had lost." So as challenging as it may be, try to keep a slight smile on your face, as contemporary scientific research agrees it can lift your mood.

WAYS TO SUPPORT YOURSELF

HUM

HUG OFTEN

DANCE TO MUSIC

BREATHE DEEPLY

WALK IN NATURE

Sherry Lynn Harris

LEARN TO MEDITATE

WATCH THE SUNRISE

TAKE A YOGA CLASS

GET YOUR HAIR DONE

COUNT YOUR BLESSINGS

RELAX BY GETTING A MASSAGE

TAKE A NAP IN THE AFTERNOON

TALK WITH YOUR SUPPORT TEAM

GO TO LUNCH WITH A POSITIVE FRIEND

WAVE AND SMILE AT PEOPLE YOU PASS

PAMPER WITH A MANICURE OR PEDICURE

BE FORGIVING OF YOURSELF AND OTHERS

GO TO THE BEACH AND WATCH THE WAVES

LAY ON THE GRASS AND LOOK AT CLOUDS

TAKE A BUBBLE BATH & listen to bubbles pop

TELL SOMEONE YOU LOVE THEM
(with no attachment to their response)

GET ADVICE ON SUPPORT PROGRAMS
(available from Social Services)

GET SOMETHING NEW FOR YOURSELF
(even just a scarf, even if it's just 'new' to you)

IMMERSE YOURSELF IN A POOL AND
LET NEGATIVITY DRAIN INTO THE WATER

BE KIND AND GENTLE TO YOURSELF

"Go Easy on Yourself – A New Wave of Research Urges" in an article from the New York Times (2/28/2011). It states "people who score high on tests of self-compassion have less depression and anxiety and tend to be happier and more optimistic." Quietly remind yourself that nobody does everything perfectly, as you embrace endeavoring to be kinder and gentler with yourself and more accepting of your limitations.

We are looking for ways to heal our whole being – body, mind and spirit. We can do so by choosing to live in a way that sustains each of these three aspects of our self. For example, the body can be supported through exercise and massage; the mind can be supported by educating oneself on what can be expected at each stage of the disease and by reading uplifting material; the spirit can be supported by walks in nature and nurturing times of silence or meditation. By finding ways to support all three aspects – body, mind, and spirit – we come into a greater sense of balance, wholeness, and healing.

One aspect of the Alzheimer's experience that can be unbalancing is that there may be times when your parent doesn't recognize you, but rather thinks that you are someone else. They can become agitated when you contradict what they believe is true. They can get angry or upset when they feel you are saying their perception of reality isn't right or you don't believe them. Instead of getting frustrated by explaining numerous times who you are, you can choose to take a mini vacation by jumping into the role of being someone else. *What?*

For instance, if your loved one mistakes you for her best friend from school, why not offer to be that person for her for a little while? You can have a lovely visit, making up stories of the old times they shared. This game can stimulate your creativity, and can turn a potentially sad experience into a fun endeavor. It's all in the way you look at it.

You can also choose to take a mini mind vacation whenever you need a break. Take time for yourself to calm and find inner peace by resting for a few minutes sitting in a private quiet corner in silence. Repeat this affirmation: "In the silence I find peace." If you have trouble relaxing into a peaceful state, try a guided visualization like those on my "Serenity Visualizations" CD, available on my website, www.Adapt2Alz.com.

Or use your imagination to picture in your mind's eye a beautiful, serene place you would like to be. It can be somewhere you have been before or you can use your creativity. See this setting in as much detail as possible. Involve all of your senses, visualizing not only what it looks like, but how relaxed it makes you feel. What are the delicious smells wafting on the wind? Is it the fragrance of a particular flower or perhaps the smell of freshly baked bread? What soothing sounds are you listening to? Perhaps you are hearing the gentle sound of a waterfall or the sweet song of birds. Picture yourself taking a bite of an exceptionally tasty treat, experiencing the flavor and texture in vivid detail. What kinds of clouds are in the sky? Are you sitting on a grassy meadow or on a sandy beach? The more you involve your imagination, experiencing details, the more peace you can create for yourself to enjoy. Time spent in this altered reality is refreshing and you will find yourself calmer and better equipped to handle the rest of your day.

A different form of altered reality is what your loved

one with Alzheimer's is experiencing. For example, many people who have lived through wartime get worried when they hear about or see news footage of war-torn areas. My cousin helped allay fears her mother had by preparing her mom a bag packed with assorted necessities. In case they had to go to the bomb shelter, she was all ready. They installed "blackout" curtains in her room and even bought her camouflage gear she could wear if she wished. When my aunt became afraid to sleep, worried that soldiers might attack in the middle of the night, my cousin told her that they were all safe because she had hired a guard to walk the perimeter of the grounds. With all of these reassurances, her mother felt very safe and "the war" ceased to be a problem.

When choosing your reality, count your blessings instead of your woes. Some people create a "Blessing Book" with their parent, listing what they are grateful for accompanied by photos or pictures you can cut out together from magazines.

I remember how frustrated I was when Mom would repeat the same thing over and over and over again. And yet years later, when she was no longer able to speak, I would have given so much just to be able to hear her voice again, and have her communicate to me with words. So be careful what you ask for and strive to appreciate whatever the current reality is.

I love the story Corrie ten Boom tells in her book *The Hiding Place*, where she and her sister were stuck in freezing cold barracks in a World War Two German concentration camp. Her sister said they must be grateful and bless their circumstances. Corrie had a hard time with this and especially couldn't see why she should bless even the pesky fleas which were all around them, but her sister insisted they should. They found out later that the reason the people in their barracks were left on their own so much, and therefore had a much easier time than all the others, was because the cruel guards didn't want to be around the fleas. It just reminds me that what we might one day consider a curse, can another day be seen as a blessing.

Answer the question "I will be happy when ____." Really think about this – when can I be happy?

The answer is "when I decide to be." So look for the good and praise it. Be grateful for what you do have. Take your parent out to eat for as long as he can enjoy it, for the day may come (as it did for us) when he can no longer figure out how to lift his body out of the restaurant booth. Enjoy long drives as often as you can, for the day may come (as it did for us) when he can no longer decipher how to climb in and out of the car. Read and sing to him and, most of all, choose to love him.

Chapter 12
Playful Ideas

"The power of imagination is infinite."
– John Muir

Thank goodness for laughter – it has eased many a difficult moment. One year when Thanksgiving dinner was over, we decided to play a rousing game of "Pass the Pigs" around the dinner table. We explained the object was to roll the two small plastic piggies like dice and score points depending on how they landed (standing up, on their back, on their snout, etc.).

Although simple, it was too hard for Mom to grasp the idea. When it came time for her first turn, she busily played with the pigs, carefully setting them in the different positions. I took her hand and showed her how to roll the piggies like dice, and then we moved on to the next player and so on, around the table.

By her next turn, Mom was again uncertain about what she was supposed to do. With all of us shouting and encouraging her to roll the piggies, she frantically looked around, knowing she was expected to do *something* with the piggies, and ended up dramatically stuffing them down her blouse! This set the whole group to laughing uproariously, and Mom grinned widely, basking in the glow of attention she received. On her next turn, again not knowing what to do with the piggies, she put them in her mouth! Again, we all laughed, retrieved the pigs, cleaned them off and passed them to the next player, while Mom beamed as if she felt she was very clever.

I couldn't help thinking how wonderful it was that we all accepted her limitations so beautifully now, and not one of us was disgusted or upset with her behavior. We all just laughed with her, happy that she could still have a good time and be a part of the fun and games.

It's for moments like this that I am truly grateful and feel all our efforts are worthwhile.

Do all you can to let your loved one know you value him as an important member of the family. Include him by inviting him to help with undemanding chores. Several uncomplicated duties which he can manage help make him feel he is contributing to the family household. Remember that simple repetition can be soothing, so he might enjoy raking leaves or sweeping the patio.

My mom loved to wipe off the kitchen counters, dry dishes and fold fresh laundry. These common, everyday tasks offer a homemaker reassuring familiarity. It can also generate a sense of accomplishment when she is still able to complete these productive tasks. When she starts having difficulty, try taking each activity one step at a time. For example, instead of asking her to set the table, give her the plates to place around the table. When that is completed, give her the napkins, then forks and so on until the setting is completed. Be sure to thank her for helping.

A great way to have playful fun together is to garden. Try planting a simple herb garden in a window box, so it's not overwhelming. You may want to let her choose the varieties of herbs. When the herbs are grown, ask which ones she'd like to use in a recipe (for example, Rosemary Chicken) and be sure to let everyone know when they are dining on the herbs she grew herself.

Several activities are both easy and fun when you release any pre-conceived ideas of what the results should be. For example, gather some long lasting flowers with sturdy stems (like chrysanthemums) and greens (like lemon leaves) and let her create a flower arrangement for the dining table. Or help her decorate a cake or cupcakes for dessert. You can give her an assortment of colored sprinkles and toppings to choose from. As long as you accept that there is no wrong way to do it, you'll both be pleased with the results.

The more you can help your parent keep their brain active, the longer they may be able to function at a higher level. The books we loved for this were the *I Spy* series. These are picture puzzles, where you try to locate familiar, common objects hidden in the photos. Each double page spread is a different theme, such as a heavenly scene of white fluffy clouds, with fanciful hidden objects to find – gold stars, angels, a unicorn and similar things. Turn the page and you discover a forest woodland scene with hidden bunnies, squirrels and deer. You can alternate finding the objects together and both be entertained for ages.

Another exercise researchers suggest as helpful in retaining brain skills is doing jigsaw puzzles. Just be sure they're not too difficult, for then they become frustrating instead of entertaining. We started with the giant 1,000 piece puzzles that Mom was quite good at, but when she started hiding the pieces in napkins and under cushions, we knew it was time to drop down to simpler puzzles. Some days she couldn't relate the picture on the box to the puzzles, but other days she could do them just fine. By continuing to simplify the number of puzzle pieces, you and your parent can enjoy sharing this activity for even several years.

When your parent is at the stage of acting more like a child, you can really have some fun with them if you allow yourself to get into the spirit. I remember talking with my girlfriend about what present to get Mom for Christmas one year. I knew that none of the things I gave her in the past would be appropriate this time. When she asked what I thought Mom would like, I haltingly admitted that I thought what she really would like was a teddy bear.

But then I cried at the thought of getting my mother – my formerly world-class executive, "I-Can-Juggle-A-Hundred-Tasks-At-Once-And-Get-Them-All-Accomplished" mother – a stuffed animal. My girlfriend talked about how much fun my mom would get out of playing with the bear and helped me see that although Mom's interests had dramatically changed, I could certainly learn to play with her at her current level. I bought Mom the teddy bear and it was just what she wanted.

As Mom "grew younger," the books I read to her were simpler and more appropriate for her "new" age. I read to her as if she were a child, with an expressive voice full of wonder at the discoveries in the book, or exaggerated concern when that was appropriate for the story. She just loved to hear them and look at the pictures, just as any child would.

When Mom and I went to the hairdresser, I would read her a children's story out loud and everyone in the whole shop would listen and enjoy it, as if hearing it new for the first time. This is a gift you can easily give from your heart.

Picture books are wonderful for the parent who is losing his ability to read. Find books that show a subject your parent is interested in. You needn't always spend much money, as oftentimes you can find just what you want at libraries or used book shops. If your father loves cars, for example, you can pick up free brochures at car dealers picturing the latest models for him to marvel over.

Playing games is a creative phase to explore with your loved one. You can play "Beauty Shop" and enjoy gently brushing her hair, trying different styles and adding colorful ribbons or fancy hair clips. You could shave your father's face, or your mother's legs, making a game of playing with the shaving cream. You can buff his nails or give her a manicure and let her choose the color she wants painted onto her nails. These days nail polish comes in almost every color, so see if sometime she would like to have something wild, like blue or purple polish for a fun change.

As your parent's level of mental acuity changes, you can adapt the games you play with them. For instance, you may be used to playing chess with your parent. When it becomes too complicated for him to remember how to move the pieces, you can switch to playing checkers. Similarly, you might start by playing Scrabble, then simplify to an easier word game like Boggle, and when that becomes too complicated, switch to large plastic alphabet letters that can be used to spell out simple words.

Play-Doh offers hours of fun and many different ways to use the product, such as making cookie dough cutouts, or rolling the dough into ropes to construct your creations. Legos are also great for constructing. Start with the regular size Legos and, when it becomes difficult for your parent to fit the pieces together, switch to the larger size. Legos are also fun to sort by colors.

Sorting games are a popular pastime because they give

your loved one a sense of control over his environment, as well as keeping his mind active. My mother loved to spend hours sorting her coins. She felt "grown up" because she was handling money, but her real enjoyment came from sorting them and then putting them into the paper holders, so she then had rolls of dimes or pennies all of the same date.

If your parent likes fishing, you could get him a tackle box containing compartments perfect for sorting lures (no hooks, of course). At the craft store, I found a plastic box with lots of compartments and packages of brightly colored beads in various shapes that Mom could sort. Your parent may enjoy stringing the beads into necklaces as well. Get plastic lanyard strings from the craft store for stringing or you can use colored shoelaces. They may even have a bead-stringing kit with all of the above items packaged together.

Look around the craft store for other items that might entertain your parent. For a long while, my mother loved the flocked posters that came with felt tip markers to color in between the lines. When her project was finished, it looked like a stained-glass window, and we would hang it up on the wall to admire it. When the markers became too difficult and messy, we switched to crayons and coloring books.

The craft store had different kits that came in their own carrying cases, a feature I was sure the caregiving staff would appreciate. One was a set of stickers that Mom could color and another a candle-making kit with cookie cutter shapes that could be pressed into wax strips to make designs. Needless to say, we didn't give her the candle wicks so there was no possibility of ever lighting the candles!

Mom's best friend thought of giving her a gigantic box of colorful stickers and a blank book that she could paste them into, offering hours of fun. A great toy for older women who spent much of their leisure time sewing is a set of old-fashioned sewing cards where you connect the dots on the picture card by "sewing" colored shoelaces through the pre-punched holes.

Your physician can give you an idea of the approximate age at which your parent is functioning, and you can purchase toys labeled as appropriate for that age. I went to the local discount stores and found items in the two to five year preschool age range. Different shapes and colors are the most important features at this phase. Our favorite was Shape N Sort. You insert the different, brightly colored plastic shapes (circle, square, star, etc.) into the box through matching openings. This is a good mental exercise for your parent and fun as well, as is a wooden tool kit for the men, complete with large wooden screws, screwdriver, wrench, hammer and pegs all in an easy-to-carry tool box.

Many adult day care centers provide guidance in helping your parent create arts and crafts projects while giving him a sense of purpose, a place to look forward to going and a chance to meet new friends and interact with them. Search the Internet under Senior Centers listed for your city. These centers will generally take your parent up until such time as he becomes incontinent and needs to wear diapers. If you're caring for your parent in your home, this is a welcome respite for several hours during the day.

Another great way to have fun together is to read old-time stories which can trigger memories of their youth. One book I love is *Dandelion Wine* by Ray Bradbury. It reminds me of simpler times, like when the author talks about a boy's need for new sneakers to start off the summer.

We feel the excitement and the imagination the boy experiences when he tentatively slips on the new sneakers, and the magic he feels that these new shoes could bring to his life. Along with the boy, we imagine that when he is wearing these very special shoes he will be able to run with the wind, like antelopes and gazelles, through the rivers and wheat fields.

Your parent will love hearing stories like these that conjure up the simpler, "wonder-full" times of the past.

Chapter 13
Musical Notes

"Music ... gives soul to the universe,
wings to the mind, flight to the imagination,
and charm and gaiety to life and to everything."
– Plato

Dr. Oliver Sacks, Professor of Clinical Neurology and Psychiatry at Columbia University, writes about the amazing therapeutic effects of music on people with Alzheimer's disease and other dementias. He states, "Music is no luxury to them but a necessity, and can have power beyond anything to restore them to themselves and to others at least for a while." Dr. Sacks describes how familiar music is the key to eliciting emotions and unlocking words that have been silent. Regarding Alzheimer's patients, Music Therapist Barbara Jacobs, M.S. states, "The benefits of music and singing, such as mood improvement and calmer behavior, often persist for hours after the music has stopped." (www.caregiver.com)

A 2009 study "confirms the well-established, positive effect music therapy has for patients with mild to moderate Alzheimer's disease." Patients listened to music they chose, over a six month period. It "resulted in significant decreases in anxiety and depression in patients. Moreover, the benefits lasted for up to two months after the music sessions were discontinued." (www.fyiliving.com/research/effect-of-music-therapy-on-anxiety-and-depression-in-alzheimers-patients/)

The reason my mom enjoys going to church so much is

to hear the music and keep time with it. Our doctor explained that music is processed by a different area of the brain than where speech is processed. This is why some people who stutter when they speak have no trouble with stuttering when they sing.

Once, ages after she had seemingly lost the ability to speak, Mom sang all the words to "How Much is that Doggy in the Window"! It was particularly meaningful to me, because we went on a road trip when I was a little girl and we sang that song over and over in the car, as it was my favorite tune at the time.

Daniel Levitin in his book *This is Your Brain on Music* states, "We tend to remember things that have an emotional component." As a result, he says people with Alzheimer's are often able to sing songs they heard during their teens, even when they can no longer remember the name of their spouse. This behavior is also well documented in people with advanced dementia. Oftentimes when Mom could no longer talk, she could still sing the words to the Lord's Prayer.

At this time I got Mom a stuffed ducky for Easter which sang the tune "Here Comes Peter Cottontail" when you squeezed it. This was most helpful when I wanted to get her to walk with me to the car, as sometimes she could dally until I wanted to pull my hair out. I would simply take her hand, start singing this tune, and take a step on every downbeat. <u>PE</u>-ter <u>PE</u>-ter <u>COT</u>-ton-<u>TAIL</u>, <u>HOP</u>-ping <u>DOWN</u> the <u>BUN</u>-ny <u>TRAIL</u>.

I tried several others that also worked like a charm at getting her to move along. From our Girl Scout days, "We are Marching to Pretoria" was a natural, as we had always walked along to that song while hiking. With "We're <u>OFF</u> to <u>SEE</u> the

WIZ-ard, the WON-derful WIZard of OZ" you can move along at a fairly swift pace. All these songs have a verbal reinforcement of moving along, such as hopping, marching or following a yellow brick road.

When Mom could no longer sing words, she still enjoyed stepping along to tunes she could hum with a distinctive downbeat for each step, such as "The Mexican Hat Dance" – DaDUM, DaDUM, DaDUM; Da DEEdily DUM de DUM. She hummed this tune over and over like a broken record until I was praying to please let her add another song to her repertoire! Be careful what you ask for, because the next song that stuck in her brain was the children's song "The WORMS crawl IN, the WORMS crawl OUT." For a year, we walked everywhere to the accompaniment of these two tunes.

Mom loved the music in church, and in particular, watching the music director, who is a gifted pianist. One day he was really belting out a song on the keyboard and Mom started exuberantly clapping. I gently tried to take her hand and hold it to quiet her (which usually worked), but this time she just wouldn't stop clapping. Everyone knew she was just having fun appreciating the music, but I was so embarrassed I could hardly bear it. Even though everyone else handled it well, I still felt quite painfully aware that my mom was acting strangely, though I was completely powerless to prevent it.

I started to cry because I felt so bad about it, when a board member whispered in my ear, "Don't worry about it. She's having a good time. She's just enjoying herself." It helped a lot to hear her say that, to have her confirm my grateful thoughts that no one was angry at me for bringing someone to church who couldn't always contain her actions.

Best of all, the platform speaker got up to talk after the

song and said, "We appreciate your enthusiastic support, no matter *what* beat of the music you are clapping to." Everyone in the congregation laughed and it totally dispelled the tension of the moment.

We attend a non-denominational church based on Christianity called "Unity" which professes that "whoever you are when you walk through the door, we accept and love you just as you are." I have attended many churches of different faiths, but never have I met a congregation that so fully embraces their teachings and demonstrates them so consistently. Many people hug my mom at church and tell her what a lovely inner light she has, what a delight she is and how happy they are to see her…and they MEAN it!

They had never known Mom before her Alzheimer's. They never knew the dynamic businesswoman, the incredibly efficient organizational genius that she was, or any of the personality traits that are usually used as a standard by society to judge a person's worth. But they know her goodness, her childlike acceptance of the world and how she sees beauty and enjoyment in the small things of life.

The other day my friend said, "You are so lucky." I thought to myself, yes, I am, but why would someone else think so?

"Why?" I asked.

"Because you still have your mother." I thought about that, and she was right. I did not have the mother I grew up with and knew, but I did have a loving mother who was still teaching me so much about life.

She was still teaching me not only patience and sacrifice and how to do the right thing, but more importantly, she was still teaching me the greatest lesson of life: LOVE.

Even though she now seldom had the ability to say recognizable words, we could still communicate on a deeper level. There was no doubt in anyone's mind when they watched us together. They could see we shared a precious and enduring love that transcended the barriers that life put before us.

Another friend came up to me after church and said she loved to watch us together and that the beauty of our togetherness brought tears to her eyes. All these words of comfort and loving, every Sunday – how they supported me. The people politely listened to Mom's nonsense words, nodded their heads and smiled, and just accepted her. What a miraculous experience to witness.

My mom was showered by love, not only from me, but by so many others there. On Mother's Day, with the choir, I sang Sinead O'Connor's song *"This is to Mother You."* Although I choked a little at the end, everyone understood, and there wasn't a dry eye in the house.

Whatever music your parent liked before Alzheimer's, they will continue to enjoy hearing. My mom always played show tunes from musicals while we were growing up, so we played those for her along with the *Reader's Digest* collection of songs from the past decades and Frank Sinatra classics. We usually have the radio tuned to the classical station so she can hear the beautiful strains of music. If your parent is going through a restless time, classical instrumental music can often help to keep her calm.

If your parent remembers how to play an instrument, encourage him to do it often. If they don't, get some maracas or a rattle they can shake in time to the music. You can even have a craft project making your own tambourines by putting dry beans between two paper plates and stapling them together. If you don't play an instrument, be sure to get yourself a percussion instrument like a shaker or a tambourine. Then the two of you can turn up the volume and have fun "rocking out" together to the beat of the music. If your parent likes to dance, join him in that activity. These ideas are fun ways to get exercise too.

Just as you would do with your children, give some thought to what television programs and movies you watch together. First of all, I recommend that you don't take your parents with Alzheimer's out to the movies. The sound systems in movie theaters these days are way too loud and disturbing to them. Also, they are likely to become extremely agitated if they see violence in the movies.

It's much better to watch TV in a room with a small light on so your loved one is aware that he's watching a television, and it's easier to recognize that it's not real. As you watch with your parent, you'll know when he can follow the story and when it's getting too complicated for him to follow, as he will most likely continually ask questions for clarification.

When movies become too long and involved to follow, switch to watching shorter shows. Variety shows of the *Lawrence Welk* type, with singing and dancing, are easier to follow than a story with a plot and many characters. My mom always enjoyed watching the Olympics, in particular the ice skating and gymnastics. We recorded these performances and she enjoyed watching them over and over, since she didn't remember seeing them and they always seemed new to her. And, of course, she enjoyed the music.

Chapter 14
Accepting Change and Moving On

"God, grant me the serenity to
accept the things I cannot change,
the courage to change the things I can,
and the wisdom to know the difference."
- *Reinhold Niebuhr*

One day while at a restaurant, I noticed a distinctive smell and guessed that Mom had lost control of her bowels. I was personally mortified when I took her to the bathroom and, for the first time, discovered that she'd had a bowel movement in her underwear. Not only did Mom seem totally unaware that she had done it, she didn't even realize there was a problem that it was there!

When we finished and she went to wash her hands, she handed me a paper towel that looked like it had something wrapped up in it. Fortunately, I didn't automatically throw it away, but looked inside. She had taken off all of her rings to wash her hands and wrapped them in the paper towel. By this time they were no longer real diamonds, but I worried about how many things must inadvertently get thrown out.

I then returned Mom to her board and care home and regretted that the lovely Hannah who was the calm, peaceful saint who cared for the residents, was no longer there. A more loving, caring individual cannot be found, and we treasured her. After a year, she returned to Europe and it was only then that we learned her story. Hannah was part of the aristocracy and quite wealthy in her own right, but had felt her life was empty and without purpose. The board and care owner, Mary, had suggested that Hannah take a year to care for others and that she would reap the rewards and satisfaction of being of service. Hannah blossomed in her chosen service and we were all the blessed benefactors.

Her replacement, however, was Emma – a stern, gruff German woman, reminiscent of all the worst qualities of my own mom's mother. When we in our family referred to my grandma, we often used one of her favorite commands: "Achtung! Everrry body into zee truck!" Stern and dictatorial, it always seemed that it was Emma's way or the highway.

We managed as best we could until the time my mom started to need diapers. Emma would meet me at the door, along with my mom, saying disgustedly, "She has been a BAD girl. She is messing her pants. *Very bad* girl." Ouch, that hurt both Mom and me.

My mom was not "bad." She couldn't help it if she no longer was in command of her bodily functions. I didn't want my sweet mother to be told she was *bad* for something she could obviously no longer be held accountable. Would you tell a baby she was bad for needing diapers? Of course not. You understand they have no concept or ability to control their bowels. Although it's always a shock when this happens to your parent, it's not something they have power over anymore, and so we must accept it and find a way to cope with it.

Mary explained we would have to get Mom to wear diapers because she was having "accidents" every day and every night, too, causing a lot of extra cleanup and washing of sheets. We knew it was going to be difficult to get her to accept diapers, but we knew we had to try or Mom wouldn't be able to stay there. Mary told me how, now, Mom would sometimes be sitting at the dining table eating and would just let go and pee all over the floor while she ate her meal. She also said that when Mom went to the bathroom, sometimes she wouldn't do it in the toilet. Yikes, this was *really scary*. And I had just taken Mom to church and out to lunch with me three days before!

We went to the store to buy grown-up diapers for Mom for the first time. Mary has such a great understanding of what made Mom happy. She asked Mom if she would like to push the shopping cart and she did. Mom had a lot of fun pushing it, just like a kid, and I would not have even thought of it! Mary also gave her a Tootsie Pop to suck on while she pushed the cart down the aisles, and Mom was thrilled.

When we got back to the board and care, it looked like Mom was ready to eat the stick from the Tootsie Pop, so I took it out of her mouth. Then I discovered that the center was not the edible candy of a regular Tootsie Pop, but pink bubble gum. I went to retrieve it out of Mom's mouth because I was worried she would swallow it. Mom did *not* want to give it up. She bit down hard on my fingernails and wouldn't let go. She was acting like an angry dog who thought I was trying to take away her bone, as she whipped her head back and forth with my fingernails clamped tightly in her teeth. As she grunted her displeasure and glared at me with anger, I felt sincerely frightened and realized with the impact of experiencing it first hand, that Mom could be a truly terrifying force to reckon with now.

At that moment, it didn't seem that there was any part of the mother I knew left. She didn't recognize me or have any knowledge of who I was or what I was doing, other than taking away something she wanted. To placate her, I quickly scraped off a part of the hard candy stuck to the gum and put it back in her mouth and disappeared into the kitchen to throw away the other remains where she couldn't find them.

It had all happened so fast, it seemed. We had been going along so well and nicely for such a long time. I knew deep down that when Mom needed help with diapers, wandering, and aggression we would need to move her again. Still, it amazes me how we can know something on an intellectual level yet manage to suppress it. The next step for Mom was an Alzheimer's facility, which I feared could be a pretty brutal reality.

When you've had the pleasure of seeing your mother in a loving home with marble bathrooms and oak floors, eating off real china with real silver and real glasses, it's hard to think that the next step is a place where they lock the doors so people can't wander off.

Mary said she would keep Mom for as long as possible, because, thank goodness, I was able to get Mom to wear the diapers. I asked Mary to let me try to get Mom to wear them by myself, but Emma said, "No, I am the one taking care of her, I will be there with you."

On the way to her room, Emma said, "I know her. She won't wear them. You will see." With such a lack of encouragement, I didn't even want Emma there. But it didn't seem I had a choice. When we started, Mom held her legs close together and wouldn't let me slip the diapers between her legs and Emma, feeling triumphantly vindicated, said, "See?"

Fortunately, Mom eventually relented and let me slip them on and fasten them. Helpful hint: When first starting with diapers, try to find the "pull-up" kind so you can tell your loved one that this is a new kind of underwear you think she might like. To the memory-impaired individual, this is not as recognizable as a "diaper" and can therefore be an easier transition. One positive – although you now need to buy diapers, at least you no longer need to buy underwear.

Now Mom's Adult Day Care program said she could not continue to attend. Mom was no longer able to figure out how to use the bathroom because of her diapers, but still insisted on trying, and they could not contend with that aspect.

I knew that when we moved Mom into a residential home, the prognosis was for just two years – but it was such a lovely two years. I couldn't imagine finding a nicer place for my mom, where she could have the privacy of her own room, surrounded by all her favorite possessions and the camaraderie of a loving staff (other than Emma) who hugged her daily and saw to her needs and comfort.

How much quieter and lovelier than the retirement center she was at before, where they woke everyone up like revile at 7 a.m. by a loudspeaker piped directly into her room. How unjust that the staff represented the intercom as a safety measure for always being able to hear your loved one cry out if they were hurt, when in reality, it was more a way of controlling them: to wake them, call them to meals and check on them without bothering to walk into their room. How Mom hated that, and how we tried (without success) to get it disconnected.

How wonderful it had been at the board and care home to know that Mom could sleep in whenever she wanted, and that the staff would always fix her breakfast when she woke up.

To know she had beautiful surroundings, so that if all she could do was look at them, you knew she was enjoying the view.

How wonderful that, instead of horrible plastic plates and glasses that seemed to make any food unappealing, Mom could eat off real china.

How sweet it was to walk in unannounced and find that the staff had just cut her a fresh peach in slices as an afternoon snack.

How scary to think that all this could disappear in the blink of an eye and that it might soon be time to move Mom to a locked Alzheimer's facility because she was wandering at night instead of sleeping and could no longer control her bowels.

When I finally was able to bring myself to ask Mary the question, "Do we have to move Mom now?" and broke down crying, how compassionate she was in her reply.

"We love your mom, and she loves us," Mary said. "I know how I would feel if it were my mom. There are some possible alternatives. We may need to hire a night nurse to watch her. We'll have to raise the rent because now we are experiencing a lot of extra work – we are changing the sheets twice a day and have to change her clothes several times a day. But you will not have to move her until we can no longer handle it. We'll manage somehow."

Relief and gratitude swept over me. At least I had some breathing space in which to locate a new home which had people specifically trained on how to handle Mom's new phases of incontinence, wandering and growing episodes of aggression.

I called my sisters and they were surprisingly supportive. They had just finished a religious retreat and said they were thinking of getting me a gift to show how much they appreciated me for caring for Mom. Who would have ever thought that a family could go through all the love we shared, then through all the distrust and pain and grief, and come out loving again on the other side? What a blessing to have them there for support. My sister Genevieve even agreed to help look for a new place for Mom, and my sister Stephanie agreed to look at Alzheimer's places where she lived. When they did not take over Mom's care when she first moved to a retirement community, they had then agreed that one of them would take over care of Mom when she needed to be placed in an Alzheimer's Special Care Unit.

At this point it had been a long ten years that Mom and I had been through together – a lot of shared fears and tears, from the first forgotten names to the last indignity of diapers. I felt really good that I lived up to her and Daddy's (and even my own) expectations of me. I was glad that I toughed it out, because it brought me a lot of pleasure to share all this love with my mom.

When someone tells me, "I can't drive with your mother in the car because she drives me crazy pointing at everything,"…then I am quietly content inside to know that I helped Mom by just listening to her and looking where she pointed when we went on drives. Acknowledging that "Oh yes, the clouds are pretty today," or "Yes, the bougainvillea looks spectacular in bloom, what a beautiful color," or "Yes, I see the plane – I wonder where they're going today."

…That I was there for her in her darkest hours of fear, when she knew her mind was slipping away and could do nothing to prevent it, like sand running out through an hourglass.

…That I held her hand as we walked along, swinging

our hands together like a couple of kids, singing "There goes Peter Cottontail, hopping down the bunny trail" or even humming with her the tune to "The worms crawl in, the worms crawl out" when that musical selection was stuck in her head.

...That I was able to release my anger at her silly gurgling over every baby, no matter how unattractive they seemed to me, and sincerely learned to enjoy the moment with her, saying "Yes, I see the baby. Isn't it a wonderful bundle of joy?"

...That we could put our heads together and pour over fitting the pieces of the puzzles together, from the 1,000 piece sets down to the 5 piece sets.

...That we could look in the picture books and have fun pointing out "Where's the angel?" or "How many stars can we count?"

...That I could see her glowing with joy, sitting in the front pew at church, bouncing her stuffed animal in time to the music, and watching her radiant face as I sang hymns to her with the choir.

Yes, the trials have been many, but so have the rewards. What an experience of growing, of understanding, of learning empathy and compassion and unconditional love. I am truly not the same person I was ten years ago when we first embarked on this journey together, but have grown into a person that I can be proud of when I look into my heart of hearts and know that I came through for my mom.

And it's a good feeling.

Chapter 15
Aggression – a Phase that Passed

"An Eastern monarch once charged his wise men to invent him a sentence which should be true and appropriate in all times and situations.
They presented him the words:
'And this too shall pass away.'"
– *Abraham Lincoln*

The Alzheimer's Association states that "people with Alzheimer's actually experience two different kinds of symptoms. The first, which are referred to as cognitive symptoms, disrupt memory, language and thinking. The second, known as behavioral and psychiatric symptoms, can cause personality changes and agitation. The chief cause of behavioral and psychiatric symptoms is the progressive deterioration of brain cells. However, medication, environmental influences and some medical conditions can also cause symptoms or make them worse." (www.alz.org)

Up to half of Alzheimer's patients can show aggressive behavior. Patients who are unable to communicate often express their discomfort from medication side-effects like constipation or nausea by becoming even more agitated and combative. *A Place for Mom* states "Perhaps the most comforting thing about Alzheimer's aggression is that, for many patients, it's a phase that will pass." (www.alzheimers.ap laceformom.com/articles/alzheimers-aggression/)

Their environment should be as non-threatening and

113

calming as possible, with no loud noises or shadows which could be misinterpreted. (www.healthcentral.com/alzheimers/c/57548/50050/agrression/2).

When your parent gets to the stage where watching television is too confusing, an aquarium is a wonderful substitute. He can enjoy watching the color and movement of the fish without the need to use more complicated reasoning, as he would if he were trying to follow a movie plot, for instance. Watching fish in an aquarium is also a good way to calm down an agitated person.

The employee at my local fish store was most helpful in assembling a small aquarium that would fit on Mom's shelf. When I explained our situation, he agreed to do everything for me, so all I had to do was fill it with water and plug it in. He even added a night light and suggested a scuba diver accessory that blew bubbles out of his snorkel so Mom would always have something to watch in the tank, even if the fish died.

It turned out neither I nor the caregivers were great at taking care of the aquarium and after repeatedly scooping out dead fish, I came up with an easier solution. We kept Mom entertained with a movie that showed brightly colored fish swimming among beautiful shades of living coral. I purchased it from the Maui Ocean Center: The Hawaii Aquarium – check with your local aquarium to see if they sell a fish movie. I often got caught up in watching the beautiful displays of color and movement while visiting, and was amazed at how calming it was.

Mom and I both needed calming on the days I came to visit. Emma, her new caregiver, would start pushing away the puzzle my mom had spent hours working on, saying it was time to put the pieces back in the box now that her daughter was here to visit. I rescued the puzzle and said I'd be happy to visit with my mom while we worked on the puzzle together. How grateful my mother was for my intervening on her behalf, as she was devastated to see all of her careful, painstaking work being so carelessly destroyed.

No matter how often I explained to Emma that people with Alzheimer's often get upset with abrupt change, she would still interrupt whatever my mom was doing, such as grabbing the coloring book and crayons away from Mom when I came to see her, telling her it was time to visit with me instead.

This day, when it was time for me to leave, Mom wanted to walk me to the front door as she usually did, but Emma didn't want to take the time to walk to the door with us and then take Mom back to her room. She told Mom to stay there with her in the room. As I said, Emma has the personality of a German drill sergeant, so with reluctance I decided it was easier to just leave rather than try to talk Emma into letting Mom walk me to the door. As soon as I left to walk out and it was clear Mom wouldn't get to walk up front with me, Mom slammed the door really hard, shaking the entire house.

I went right back and while Emma complained, "See how she is?" I walked up to Mom and said in my sternest impression of her mother's accented voice, "DOAN SLAM DOOR!" When she looked at me, I could see her confusion and anger. I could also see that she didn't really have any understanding at that moment of who I was. I immediately realized that I should not scold mom, knowing that patients respond better to a calm and reassuring voice. So as the moment of anger passed, I said in the fun voice we used when playing together, "You want to walk me to the door?" She nodded yes. "OK, you walk me to the door, no problem. You have problem? I no have problem. *No problem.*"

I know that environment can affect behavior, so I wondered how much of the aggression Mom was showing was brought on by Emma's dictatorial attitude. I asked Mary if it was possible to get a different caregiver, but she was not ready to do that.

Mom had a hard time adapting to diapers. One reason was that Emma was not experienced in changing adult diapers and clearly didn't want to have that experience. As the upset caregiver increased her anger and animosity toward my mother, Mom responded, becoming more obstinate and angry herself.

Mary came to me asking that I take Mom to the doctor because she was becoming aggressive and we needed medication to calm her down. Mary went with me to the appointment three days later. While we waited in the waiting room, she told me that Mom's abilities and functioning had deteriorated the past couple of months. Mom used to spend hours playing with puzzles and she understood that the picture on the front of the box was how you put the puzzle together. Now Mary said she didn't even understand which pieces go with which puzzles – it was all the same to her.

Mary said it started off that about once a week Mom would get aggressive when they tried to get her to do something she didn't want to do, like take a shower. Now it had progressed to where it was a problem every day. When I suggested that we hire someone other than Emma, she said the problem was not just with Emma, but with everybody.

Mom now weighed 208 pounds, and she could be quite

adamant and forceful when she wanted things her way. That's the difference between an older person who acts like a baby and a real baby – a couple hundred pounds can really pack a wallop! Still, it seemed so unlike my mom. I didn't want to accept the reality that she had changed so much that she could actually physically harm someone.

Our immediate need was to control Mom's combative outbursts. Since Mom's regular doctor was out of town, another doctor prescribed Haldol®, which I later learned is an anti-psychotic drug usually used to control hallucinations and delusions, used in this case for anti-anxiety. It was so potent that soon it was putting Mom into a vegetative state.

When Mom's regular doctor returned the following week he agreed that Haldol was too strong for Mom and recommended Risperdal®. Compared to Haldol, Risperdal has "been found to be somewhat more effective in reducing behavioral problems" although it "has **not** been approved for use in dementia patients by the FDA." (http://alzheimers.aplac eformom.com/articles/alzheimers-aggression/) He said using Risperdal as an anti-anxiety medication could help Mom to get a proper amount of sleep which should help reduce her outbursts of anger and aggression.

Mom was also taking one of the cholinesterase inhibitor medications most commonly given to delay the progression of symptoms of Alzheimer's: Aricept. Our doctor said at this point Aricept, most often used to improve brain function in the early to middle stages of Alzheimer's, would no longer help Mom.

I asked the doctor about alternative natural therapies like Ginko Biloba. He said we could give it to her, as it had been shown to help in some cases, and he also suggested

Vitamin E. I was surprised and pleased we had a doctor who was open to non-traditional medicines. In the *Encyclopedia of Mental Disorders* I read, "A naturopathic approach to Alzheimer's includes supplementing antioxidant vitamins (vitamins A, E and C) in the patient's diet. Botanical supplements that have been said to improve cognitive function include an extract made from *Gingko Biloba.* Gingko Biloba Extract (GBE) is the most frequently used herbal medicine in Europe and has been approved by the German Commission E for dementia-related memory loss. Gingko extract is thought to work in a manner similar to the cholinesterase inhibitors." (http://www.minddisorders.com/A-Br/Alzheimer-s -disease.html) At present, controversy remains in the United States over the effectiveness of GBE: some studies show cognitive improvement in patients while other studies do not.

With the help of different anti-anxiety medication, supplements of vitamin E and Ginko Biloba, our hope was that Mom could stay in residential care a while longer. Unfortunately, we soon had another setback when I received a horrible phone call. Mom was "writhing on the floor in pain" and I had to come and take her to the emergency room at the hospital. At that time, I was two hours away working at a convention, so I had to contact Mom's medical provider by phone and get approval for Mary to take her to the hospital until I could arrive.

Anyone who has dealt with a large insurance company has horror stories, and this is just one more. I felt so helpless as I was transferred from department to department with no one offering any assistance until after almost an hour I ended up back where I started. When the first person again heard the description of my mother "writhing in pain on the floor," he recognized my story, took pity on my now distraught state and told me to have Mary take Mom to Emergency.

When I arrived at Emergency two hours later, the staff still had not seen my mother. They were waiting on a urine sample, actually expecting us to get it from my mom. *Not* realistic. I explained this to the staff, and also that Mom could become violent, as she had finally "had it" with Emma and released all of her pent up fury, frustration, pain and rage by walloping Emma with the considerable force of her 200 plus pounds. Based on the assumption that Mom's problem could be an infection, the emergency room doctor prescribed antibiotics without an examination.

When Mom was no better the next day, Mary and I again had to take her to Emergency. There are times like these when it's very important to follow your instincts. When you strongly feel that something is wrong, you need to pursue getting the situation rectified. This time we *insisted* she be examined, and it was only then that we discovered Mom had a raging yeast infection. For anyone who hasn't experienced a yeast infection, it's very painful and itches so much it practically drives you out of your mind. It's a condition that is *aggravated* by antibiotics. If we had not insisted on the examination, we wouldn't have found the real problem. Thankfully, the doctor prescribed the correct medication and Mom was on her way to recovering.

Mom had, of course, alienated Emma by "decking" her with her tremendous punch, and it was clear that Emma could not, and would not, cope with changing Mom's diapers. Not surprisingly, Mary asked me to find Mom another home. We needed a place where the caregivers knew how to care for an Alzheimer's elder in diapers and in the aggressive stage. Most importantly, we needed caregivers who were further trained and competent in providing the proper care for people with Alzheimer's.

According to the *Encyclopedia of Mental Disorders*, "The middle stage of AD [Alzheimer's Disease] is the point at which the behavioral and psychiatric symptoms that are so stressful to caregivers often begin— the agitation, wandering, temper outbursts, depression and disorientation." Agitation "may result from the changes in the patient's brain tissue, or it may be a symptom of depression associated with Alzheimer's disease." (www.minddisorders.com/A-Br/Al zheimer-s-disease.html)   It usually occurs in the middle stages and passes on when the patient enters the later stages of the disease.

If you've been caring for your loved one in your home, you need professional advice when they enter the aggressive stage. You need to understand and accept that it's not fair to you or the rest of your family to have someone who is uncontrollably violent in your home. A specialized Alzheimer's care facility employs people who are trained in distracting an aggressive patient and redirecting their thoughts so that violence is often avoided. I was in despair that I wouldn't find any place that I'd be happy moving Mom into, and was worried that it was time to look into Medi-Cal (read government assistance) and a nursing home. After two whole years of relative stability, I felt all the responsibilities and worries crushing down on me again.

I went to an elder law attorney, desperate for direction on my next move. He said if I didn't move Mom to a skilled nursing facility when it was obvious her current care home could no longer meet her needs, I could be open to charges of elder abuse. Me? Abusing my mommy? All I wanted to do was the right thing. I was very scared. I became convinced that I needed the lawyer to complete the Medi-Cal application forms to be sure Mom would be approved for government assistance. Even though the paperwork the lawyer asked me to sign had all kinds of dire stipulations saying the firm could not be sued, and the fee was $500 per hour, I signed because I didn't see that I had an alternative. (Bad choice – I suggest you don't do that).

I toured the locked Alzheimer's nursing homes and even found a good one that didn't smell and seemed the most acceptable. Even so, I couldn't see moving my mom from her private room of lace curtains, rose trimmed wallpaper and a dining room with real china into the stark sterility of two hospital beds in a shared room.

Then I remembered Nancy Wexler, the geriatric care manager I went to for advice when I needed to move Mom from the retirement community. It was she who had told me about the alternative care Mom could get in a board and care home and who directed me to the perfect place for Mom two years ago. She could tell from my voice when I called that I was riding the edge of frustration and terror and arranged for me to come in that very day to see her.

When Nancy told me I deserved a purple heart for all the wonderful care I had been giving my mom, I broke down in tears. I so terribly needed someone to affirm that I was doing a good job, and here was an expert acknowledging that she understood how difficult it was, and that I was doing the absolute best under the circumstances Mom and I were facing. I sobbed out my fears and it was a wonderful release.

Nancy told me I should *not* be paying a lawyer to

complete the Medi-Cal forms for me. Instead, I should find the absolute best place to take care of my mom for as long as funds existed. What places were these? What alternatives did I have? I wasn't aware that I had any.

She explained that I did not have to take Mom to a "skilled nursing facility" (nursing home) as the next step. Other residential care homes had people who were fully trained on how to deal with incontinence, aggression, dementia and hospice care. These were facilities who were qualified by the government to give dementia and hospice care.

What was hospice care? I wasn't familiar with this term. At the end of life, hospice care enables your loved ones to stay in their home while specially trained professionals and volunteers ease their pain and provide comfort and dignity, as well as emotional, social and spiritual support. The team has specialized knowledge of medical care including pain management to improve the quality of your loved ones' last days. This seemed far less traumatic than putting my mom in the hospital, particularly as Mom had signed a living will specifically stating we were not to use any "heroic" measures to prolong her life, but rather to "let nature take its course."

It's important to know that once a patient is hooked up to life support, it is legally very complicated to take it away. The best approach is to keep all documentation in the patient's file and discuss it ahead of time with the doctor that you specifically do *not* want CPR, feeding tubes, etc. (heroic measures). You also need a "Do Not Resuscitate" (DNR) form or a POLST form for any paramedics who might be called in an emergency, and it's a good idea to tape a copy of this to the wall over your loved one's bed. (See additional details in Chapter 3 "Putting Affairs in Order;" Forms in Appendix 1.)

Nancy said she had just visited a brand new, state-of-the-art Alzheimer's Special Care Unit which had recently opened. They used all of the most recent research ideas, such as interacting with animals and children. They were experts in helping to control aggressive behavior by "redirecting" the attention of the Alzheimer's patient, rather than by using medication.

The Alzheimer's facility had many of these "redirection" tools placed along the walls. They were used to change the attention of agitated people from what they were upset about to something else, such as pushing a button to ring a doorbell, or moving a shape to fit into a cutout position on a board. My favorite was a telephone that they could pick up and hear music and a talking voice on the other end. So many times people with Alzheimer's want to use the phone, but can't remember how. This device seems to calm their mind and make them happy that, from their perspective, they can still use a telephone – an action they performed frequently when they were well.

I was concerned that this facility was financially out of the range of what we could pay. Nevertheless, I took the brochures to see just what "state-of-the-art" could be and decided I ought to go see it for myself.

Wow! What a place! Like many others, my mom's aggression most often manifested when she was forced to take a shower or bath. Mom never was one for showers her whole life, often preferring a daily swim or a sponge bath. I could understand that her fears were justified from the time my sister and I gave her a shower after a swim. Although we thought we were being careful, Mom slipped on the slick floor and fell hard. I was so upset by this that I never again insisted she take a shower when she was with me.

However, cleanliness is really important and necessary for good health. One of the reasons we moved Mom from the retirement community to assisted living was because Mom was no longer able to take showers by herself and she was beginning to smell. (Obviously not what you want for your loved one.)

Bathing is one of the most common issues that can trigger aggression. Most elderly go through the fear of bathing at some time as they are quite understandably afraid of falling. You can help allay their fears by installing one or two secure handlebars in the shower and a sturdy shower chair – obtained from a hospital supply store. In addition, get one of the flexible hand-held shower hoses so they can sit on the chair and easily direct the water spray. If your parent bathes herself, be sure you test the water temperature so she doesn't scald or freeze herself. The Alzheimer's Store (www.alzstore.com) sells an anti-scalding device that you can easily attach to the faucet. If your loved one is no longer capable of bathing herself, these items are a big help to you in accomplishing the job of bathing with the least amount of fuss.

When my mom would say she didn't need a shower, I'd bring over her life-like baby doll and say, "We need to wash the baby. Will you go in the shower with the baby so we can wash her?" When suggested in this way, Mom was happy to oblige.

Allow yourself to accept that they don't need a shower every day unless they have odor problems. Always be sure they have a full shower or bath at least once or twice a week. In between shower days you can keep them fresh with a sponge bath or wet wipes, which is easier and faster.

If you have a parent who is uncomfortable about being naked, you can wrap a large bath towel around her and fasten it with Velcro or a clip or safety pin. The last of her clothing can be removed from under the towel. Then she can step into the shower with the towel still on and you can wash and rinse under the towel, thereby preserving her sense of dignity.

At this stage, my mom was past being willing to take a shower because she was afraid of falling. This facility provided the perfect answer – a large no-slip floor that drained so that the whole room was a walk-in shower with no ledge to climb over.

Mom used to love baths, but now she was afraid to climb in and out of the bathtub. They also seemed to have a great solution for taking a safe bath, with a miraculous bathtub with a sliding side. This tub has a "seat" at chair level and your parent can simply sit down in the tub as she would sit on a chair. Then she swings her legs into the tub, the side comes up and hydraulically seals to prevent the water from leaking out, and the bathtub is rapidly filled. Very easy, and much less likely to have any problems slipping and falling, or being unable to get up and out of the bathtub!

In addition, the "spa" room was so pleasantly decorated – including aromatic candles – that it was very inviting. It would take the professionals a while to get Mom used to the new system, but the point is that they caringly did.

Combined with the caring, qualified staff, the formal dining room where they used real china, the three foot deep swimming pool for water exercises (a favorite pastime of my mom's) and the lovely grounds which feel like you're strolling through the park, how could I ever want for a better place to care for my special mom? I was even able to select the room with the best view for her, overlooking the garden and a slope of hillside covered with beautiful pine trees. So what if the money runs out? When it did, she would be that much farther along in her dementia and maybe by that time, it wouldn't matter so much that she needed to be in a Medi-Cal facility.

After all, a lovely oak front door which was locked was a far cry from seeing a bolted steel door with a peephole window in it. A shared room with an armoire, matching bedspreads and a beautiful view was far preferable to a stark hospital bed. A "country kitchen" area where my mom could "play" at cleaning the counters, one of the things she still liked to do at my house, was far more encouraging to keep her at her present skill level.

I particularly liked all the areas set aside for the residents to interact with one another, like living room settings with comfortable chairs and glowing fireplaces. Even though my mom rarely uttered a distinguishable word now, and mostly babbled, she did it with such charm that I was sure she would make friends here. Mom had always been very sociable, and she had limited chances to socialize in the board and care home for the past two years, because the new caregivers didn't speak much English and the other residents didn't want or weren't capable of making much conversation. I was hopeful Mom would glow with all the added attention. After all, back at the retirement center, she was the belle of the ball at the weekly dances.

When I asked Mom after we toured the Alzheimer's Special Care Unit if she would like to live there, she emphatically lit up with a big smile and pantomimed that she wouldn't walk through the door to go back outside, indicating that she didn't want to leave.

I was relieved to find such a lovely way to solve the problem of Mom's aggression. (After less than a year at this Alzheimer's care facility, my mom was no longer aggressive and we were then able to move her to a less expensive alternative.)

Even though Mom was happy to move to her new home, keep in mind that each time a person with Alzheimer's must adjust to new surroundings, his skills in coping diminish. He's confronted with a lot of different situations and, due to the impaired functioning of his brain, it's very difficult to learn new things. It's important for you to visit him often right after a move so that, just like a child, you reassure him that you know where he is and how to find him.

For those who have a hard time knowing what to say to your loved one, you can always visit during "movie time." Fred Astaire movies and old musicals like *Singin' in the Rain* and *Oklahoma* are popular because even if the residents can't follow the story, they enjoy the music and dancing. Facilities usually show movies in a community room and you can sit next to your parent in the dimmed light and watch the movie together, sharing the experience, relieved of the need to talk. You may want to try holding her hand for a while, or putting your arm around her.

Making emotional connections with your loved ones has so many benefits. Not only does it give them the closeness so important to humans in general, it can also slow down the progression of Alzheimer's. According to a Senior Health News article, a study led by Johns Hopkins and Utah State University researchers suggests that "a particularly close relationship with caregivers may give people with Alzheimer's disease marked edge over others in retaining

mind and brain function over time." (http://www.medindia.net
/news/Emotional-Closeness-With-Caregivers-Can-Slow-Alzhei
mers-Progression-Study-55210-1.htm#ixzz1XIhJVtmS)

Remember when you were young and were sick and maybe even scared? For me, it always seemed less painful and at least a little bit better if my mom was there with me. It's your *actual physical presence* that can be of real comfort to your loved one. Choose to be there for her.

Chapter 16
Does She Recognize You?

"The trick is in what one emphasizes.
We either make ourselves miserable,
or we make ourselves happy.
The amount of work is the same."
– Carlos Castaneda

On my first visit to see Mom, five days after the move to her new home at the Alzheimer's facility, I was surprised that she didn't seem to recognize me like she always had before. I think perhaps the newness of all the changes and the fact that she was now around so many new people adversely influenced her ability to distinguish my "difference" from the crowd.

Even though Mom didn't want to give up the baby doll she was carrying in one hand or the teddy bear she carried in the other in order to take my hand for a walk, I accepted this in stride, and just put my arm around her as we walked down the halls together.

Since there was no place safe to take her really, it was a comfort to have a nice large place to walk around, with many pictures on the walls to look at and many treasures in the glass-fronted cabinets to admire together.

When the weather was warm we could walk in the lovely gardens, but it was too cold to do that at this time of year.

I was at a bit of a loss as to what to do with her, so I

rummaged through the few toys and books I had brought, and pulled out one of her favorites – a picture book of Anne Geddes photographs of precious babies.

I went to the front desk to retrieve one of the two pairs of Mom's glasses I had left in their care. During my original tour, the director pointed out that they kept track of the residents' glasses for them, keeping them in a special cupboard at the front desk.

As so often happens, the reality didn't match the original presentation. The person who had the key to the cupboard was out of the building and wouldn't return for another hour and a half.

Only then did I realize that I would have been better off keeping a pair of Mom's glasses with me so she would at least be assured of having them when I was visiting.

I was disappointed, knowing Mom couldn't see the pictures as well without her glasses, but we nevertheless made our way to one of the comfortable sitting areas, where she indicated that she liked the fire in the fireplace.

We snuggled the baby doll, the teddy bear and ourselves together into the couch. Nearby a bird brightly chirped in its cage and we had fun taking turns imitating the bird's calls.

We turned the pages of the book and Mom's face lit up with happiness to see the sweet baby photographs. She clapped her hands with joy when we turned to a page with clusters of two and three babies grouped together like sunflowers. She counted the groups, pointing to them and correctly saying "two" and "three." It was very encouraging that she got this right.

For a little variety we walked down to the "Country

Kitchen," one of the areas where residents can fix a simple snack, like toast, and socialize together. For women who were homemakers, this is an important place where they feel they belong, and encourages them to retain their kitchen skills by using them.

The staff was in the process of installing the television cable, so it wasn't working yet. We sat on the couch and I was delighted when Mom looked up and noticed our reflections in the expanse of the blank TV. She combed her fingers through her hair to make it look better. For a moment, as we gazed at our happy reflections, it was like old times when we didn't need to talk, but were just happy sitting side by side next to each other.

We went back to looking at the book and by the end she was counting the babies correctly, getting beyond the "threes" to include "four" and "five." She even took a stab at reading some words on the room's easel, and got several of them correct.

Even though I cried when I left, in retrospect, several things had happened while we were visiting together that I could hold on to as being positive.

On the other hand, for the first time during our visits, she spent a long time being distracted, just playing with the baby doll, not remembering I was there.

She smoothed her dolly's dress and kissed her nose. I missed her doing these things with *me*.

Sometimes you just need to give up looking at the positives and feel the grief and the pain.

On the way home I wrote this poem as my way of trying to cope with our changing circumstances:

Sherry Lynn Harris

My Missing Mom

Sweet, sweet soul within your breast,
Tell me how to love you best.
Is there a way
to reach your mind?
Where you are now,
is there space or time?

I know there's no worry, no shame, no stress;
No guilt or concerns:
just the touch of my caress.
You're gone from me now, to a place far away.
Can't you come back,
for a while, and play?

I know I'm the Mommy now, you are the child.
I'll treasure your trust, knowing all the while,
You cherished and cared for me
from the day I was born;
I'll do so for you now,
though my heart be torn.

In your infinite wisdom and patience you saw
Not the imperfect me, but a child of God.
Now you no longer talk,
or look at me much,
But still we communicate
to each other through touch.

My soul reaches out to shield you with love,
And I trust you are safe with the angels above.
While your body still lingers,
we can still at least touch:
I can show you I'm grateful,
and love you so much.

The following week they called to say Mom was having trouble getting around and to please bring her a walker. When I arrived the next day with the walker, Mom was nowhere to be found. She wasn't in her room or any place I looked, and with my heart in my dry mouth, I approached the front desk and gingerly asked if they knew where she was.

"Oh yes," they replied. "Everyone went on an outing to the Griffith Park Observatory. They should be returning soon...would you like to wait?"

Relief washed over me in a palpable wave, knowing Mom was safe.

Then I was hit with a poignant disappointment – I was the one who had always taken her on outings before. Less than a week before she wasn't even able to climb into my car, the day before they suggested I bring a "walker" to help her get around, and today she was doing so well they took her on a long expedition. My head was spinning, unable to take in the seemingly conflicting ideas of Mom's state at last week, versus last night, versus today. How could I keep up with her fluctuating condition?

In a daze, I drove to my counselor's office. As usual, I was perfectly fine when we started talking, but as I continued to relate my recent experiences with Mom, I broke down and cried with the sadness of grief in losing even more of Mom's awareness of me.

I asked, "How can I answer the question most often posed to someone caring for a loved one with Alzheimer's... "Does she still recognize you?""

My counselor helped me come up with a good answer to that painful question, so that it would no longer catch me off-guard, wondering how to respond now that the unvarnished truth was too awful an admission to share. We decided I could voice my perception of the truth by saying, "The only way I can answer that question is to say that she always seems happy to see me."

Of course, the pain and the shame was that she was always happy to see anyone. It no longer seemed that I was any different from anyone else. In fact, she seemed to give a brighter smile to some of the other caregivers, which she had no doubt spent more time with recently.

I realized that since Mom now had trouble figuring out how to get into my car, it didn't seem likely that she would be able to come to my house for Christmas morning. My aunt Min quietly but firmly pointed out that it was time to realize that Mom's days of traveling were over.

The pit of my stomach felt empty and hollow and I felt myself growing smaller, diminishing. Min added that she didn't feel up to making the drive out to our home for Christmas morning either. I was just hit with the idea that maybe my mom wouldn't be able to join us, and here my aunt was saying she couldn't come either. What would we do? My whole Christmas was disintegrating before my eyes, spiraling down to just the three of us (me, my husband and child) trying to cheer one another up, with no one else to exclaim over the presents, no one else to share the joy.

I didn't see any way out of this dilemma, since Min was starting to show signs of Alzheimer's herself, and I figured she probably didn't feel competent any longer to make the forty minute drive from her house to ours. Under the circumstances, I couldn't very well insist she come, but I was devastated at what the loss of both her and Mom's presence would do to our traditional Christmas morning celebration.

The fear that I might soon have to start this caregiving process all over again with my aunt was more than I could bear alone.

With a heavy heart, I poured out my fears to my counselor, hoping beyond hope that she could offer some help. To my surprise and delight, she had two very good suggestions. The first was to suggest to my aunt that if the drive was the reason she didn't want to come, she could spend the night at our house on Christmas Eve. We would pick her up and return her to her house after the presents and breakfast Christmas morning.

The second suggestion was that we make some change in our regular Christmas morning routine so it allowed me to feel more in control of the situation. It could be something as small as serving a different fruit or juice for Christmas breakfast. We discussed taking a walk with the dog first thing in the morning. We have some lovely hiking trails above our house and we could even sing Christmas carols as we walked, giving the neighbors below a treat if anyone were listening at that hour.

I felt a tremendous weight lifting off my shoulders and a peace settling around me, knowing that I didn't have to be a victim of my circumstances, but could actually exert some control over the situation.

I thankfully called my aunt and explained we'd be happy to pick her up and drive her and she gladly agreed to come over to share Christmas with us. A cry of relief lightened my heart as I allowed her comforting words to soothe me.

After all, the new facility was serving a Christmas dinner with all the families the night before Christmas Eve and that would be our "quality time" with Mom. The day arrived, and Corey, Dan and I went with happy hearts to visit, taking our gifts simply held in gift bags as Mom could no longer unwrap packages. While we waited for dinner, we played a game of reindeer tiddlywinks, which kept us all entertained, trying to pop the reindeer into the Christmas box.

It was lucky we brought a diversion, as my first look at Mom was a shock indeed. The staff had tried to put makeup on Mom, and she looked like a clown, with dark pointed eyebrows painted on and a lipstick gash slashed across her mouth in bright red. I quickly blotted Mom's lipstick, trying to make it conform more to the shape of her mouth, and rubbed off most of the offending eyebrow pencil, so that once again she bore a resemblance to the mother I knew and loved.

My son Dan was having an even harder time adjusting to Mom's drastically altered condition, and we stepped out to walk down the hall a moment to collect ourselves. My son no longer visited his grandma except for holidays like Christmas (because of his earlier traumatic experience when she didn't recognize him). I told Dan how much I appreciated his being there to help me through this difficult time; that I didn't know it would be this bad, and that in all likelihood I'd never ask him to come and do this again. With this assurance, he calmed down and we returned to the dinner table. I was immensely grateful that they were serving wine, and used it to fortify myself.

We were used to seeing Mom at the board and care home with only five other residents. My usual routine was to call each person by name as I went around the dining table, giving each one a special hug and kiss. I was surprised by how disconcerted we were to see so many old people sitting in a big dining room, and by the amount of loud noise all the people created.

I brightly talked to Mom as usual, but it was clear that she had trouble following what I was saying. I held her hand, which elicited some response. Her eyes briefly cleared with a dawning understanding that I was there, before they drifted off again. I couldn't help but notice that her occasional brightest smiles were for the other members of the staff, and not for us.

The dinner was prime rib and I was somewhat surprised that the staff had not cut Mom's meat into bite-size pieces. I proceeded to do so, and was again surprised to see her toy with her fork and finally lift a piece of food to her mouth with her hands. This was definitely new behavior and indicated another loss of her dwindling abilities to fend for herself.

Mom's face looked thinner and prettier, but now I wondered if maybe it was because she wasn't getting enough to eat. I put the fork in her hand and guided it to her mouth and asked, "Do you remember how to eat with a fork?" Her response was to insert the fork way into her mouth, practically down her throat. I quickly snatched it back, amazed that she didn't choke and gag.

Okay, I said to myself, this doesn't need to be bad or traumatic – it's just like feeding a baby. I tried feeding Mom a bite-sized piece of meat, and she meekly opened her mouth, accepted the food and chewed it. It seemed that she wanted to be fed and was happier when I did so.

I asked a staff member if they were aware that Mom no longer appeared able to feed herself. She said she would inform the staff and they sent a nice girl over to feed Mom while we were at the table.

When I brought Mom to this new facility three weeks ago, she was in strong physical health. Now she had trouble walking and eating, and no longer recognized me.

I knew you should expect Alzheimer's patients' skills to diminish whenever you move them. Change of any kind is particularly hard on them as they cannot make new pathways of connections in their brain to learn new things. Nevertheless, this Alzheimer's Special Care Unit was such a beautiful place, the people were so kind and loving, and they handled Mom's incontinence and diapers with ease (unlike her last home). Here Mom had much more activity and interaction with other people. I hoped that her communication skills might improve since so many people talked with her.

I knew that moving Mom here was the best alternative available, but each step down in her abilities was painful to me. When we left the board and care and I gave one last hug goodbye to each of the other residents, they all said they hoped Mom could be helped at her new home. I answered that there was always hope, and that we had to continue to hope, because sometimes that's all we can do.

Even with the advice of my counselor, it still remained stressful for me to answer the question, "Does she still recognize you?" I decided that I needed to change the way I felt about it. While this question is "okay" when you can still say yes, it becomes quite difficult to answer when it's no longer true. You don't want to admit it to *yourself*, let alone anyone else. But I found it took out the sting when I altered my attitude and realized that it's not the most important thing.

The fact that my mom's eyes still lit up with delight when she saw me – this was the positive I held on to. She may not have known I was her daughter, but she knew I loved her and she returned my love. This was what was important.

So when people asked, "Does she still recognize you?" I answered, *"I choose to believe that she does."*

Chapter 17
If You Only had One Word: "YES"

"A pessimist sees the difficulty in every opportunity;
An optimist sees the opportunity in every difficulty."
– *Winston Churchill*

When does the guilt of not visiting outweigh the benefits of seeing your loved one? This is a personal decision that must be made by each individual. Now that it had been 14 years into my mother's Alzheimer's journey, and Mom sometimes seemed closer to her daily caregivers than to me, I sometimes curtailed my visits to twice a month, instead of weekly. Yes, it was hard at times to remember that this frail shell of a body was my mother. But then there were the wonderful glimmers of recognition, which were the reward for continuing to honor my mother by regularly visiting her.

Yesterday, her eyes would drift off into space. I used to think the TV caught her attention, but when we turned it off, it made no difference. But then she would look at me and her eyes would clear and it seemed as if she really saw me for a while. I would talk to her then, reminding her of good times we shared over the years.

Even though it had been four years now since she was able to communicate through speech, I was convinced she could still understand, and was rewarded occasionally with the one word she still could say: Yes.

If you had just one word to remember, isn't that a good, positive word? "Yes." I would of course love her to say it when you talked about something very dear to your heart, such as, "I'm your daughter Sherry, remember?" "Yes." That would be a wonderful comfort. But don't expect too much.

I asked Mom if she remembered when she planted the 100 eucalyptus trees that lined our home's driveway.

"Yes."

I can only imagine the time and effort she put into that project. But she absolutely knew what I was talking about. I took the story and related it to me, such as when Mom and I planted the lower driveway with pine trees. Did she remember how every Christmas we would walk down the driveway together to pick out our very own Christmas tree? They looked so small in the big outdoors, but every year when we hauled the tree up to the house, we had to cut more off the top to fit it through the door. "Yes," she remembered.

If you didn't spend the time with your loved one making the effort to reminisce about all the precious times, would your loved one eventually lose these memories? I know they would not be as clear or as poignant in my own mind.

One often wonders – if I were the one with Alzheimer's, what would I want? My aunt Min always said she would rather die. But now the time was here. She was 73 and facing the onslaught of memory loss with Alzheimer's. She was scared, but still wanted to go on.

As for me, I would want to be taken care of as lovingly as my mom was, until such time as I no longer enjoyed it. Even though it had been 14 long years now, my mom really has had a pretty good time throughout most of it. When she moved into the retirement community, she hated the change of losing her independence, but this was mitigated by things she loved – the social aspects of visiting with friends, the drives through the countryside, the weekly dances, the piano recitals and especially celebrating all the holidays.

Mom loved all of the arts and crafts projects involved with the holidays, from making handmade Valentines to creating Christmas cards.

She had a very hard childhood, living through the depression with a foreign-born mother whose husband died when Mom was seven. Her mother was bitter about being left to fend for herself with three small children to support, and had no love or comfort left within her to give the children. So now Mom really enjoyed being taken care of like a little girl. There were times we would see her skipping, as she regressed; times when I was sure she was secretly pleased to be hand-fed like a baby. How she loved to get hugs and cuddles, living out the fantasy dreams she had as a child.

Why would I want to deprive her of that? Did I cry? Of course. But I also tried to dwell on each positive thing when it happened, and hold those thoughts foremost in my mind. There were things at every stage to be grateful for, times when *your* heart also says "Yes." Try to find the good in each moment, and don't wait until the stage is past to appreciate them. Try to remember that when your parent is asking you the same question over and over again until you think you have to scream, in the future when she cannot talk at all, you will treasure even just one word.

Join your parent in the discovery of their second childhood. Color with them. Do puzzles with them. Skip with them. Sing with them. Even now, after 14 years, I sang the notes of the Mexican Hat Dance yesterday and my mother joined in humming. Treasure these little miracles, and your life will be as full as it can be.

Chapter 18
Non-Verbal Communication:
The Puppy Theory

"Perhaps the most important thing we bring
to another person is the silence in us...
the sort of silence that is a place of refuge,
of rest, of acceptance of someone as they are.
Silence is a great place of power and healing."
– Rachel Naomi Remen

There were times when I thought I had it all under control...Times when I thought it was enough just to be with Mom and know that she was happy...Times when I counted my blessings that I had this much of her left to hold onto, and to savor every smile, every time her eyes lit up with recognition that it was *me* she was happy to see.

And then there were times when I poignantly rested my head on her shoulder as we both gazed into the eyes of the stuffed animal in her lap, and the shared moment reminded me of how it used to be, before the disease. How I could always talk with my mom about anything that bothered me...and how she would always listen.

I thought about my new puppy and how precious he was to me...How we bonded with each other, how we connected with each other in such a deep way that I didn't even notice that he wasn't talking verbally to me. He sure was a good listener.

So I evolved my puppy theory. If I was so close with

my dog, who was unable to speak to me, I should be able to be just as close or closer to my mom. I really liked that thought. So many people think that to be close to another, you have to spend eons of time discussing and sharing your ideas and values. And yet, here I was so close to an animal who never uttered a word of English.

Similarly, my mother no longer talked. The way I looked at my pet let him know I loved him. I could look at my mother the same way, with love in my eyes, and she could still return the love to me, tenfold, in just a look.

I could hug my pet to let him know his presence was treasured…Even more so could I hug my mom, and she hugged back…Heartfelt, comforting hugs of reassurance and protection, of love and even sharing. I could pet my dog to let him know how much I cared for him and about him…Just as I could hold my mother's hand and stroke it to communicate how much she still meant to me, and always would.

In all these nonverbal ways we were still able to communicate and share and bond on a deeper level than the sometimes superficiality of conversation. And while most of the time I was serenely accepting of these gifts, there were times when I remembered her as she was – my vibrant, healthy mother, so beautiful and intelligent and compassionate. How well I learned from her, especially the compassionate aspect.

Listen to your intuition – that small voice inside – and act on what it tells you to do. Many people hear this voice, but they tend to ignore or discount it, dismissing it as their imagination or worrying that the ideas are outrageous, or just plain wrong. Although your parent may no longer be able to converse with you, they may still be able to understand you, just on a different level.

Especially when your loved one can no longer talk, it's so important to pay attention and train yourself to listen for the guidance of your intuition. So many times when I got the impression that my mom was thirsty, I would offer her a drink and she would gratefully gulp it down as if she had been longing for it, and reward me with a big smile. This is an easy way for you to practice listening to your "inner voice" as there may be outer signs that help to guide you, such as your parent licking her lips or opening and closing her mouth.

Start practicing your intuition while your parent can still nod yes and no, and you'll be amazed at how often your "guesses" at what she wants are correct. For example, if she is staring at her reflection in the mirror, ask if she would like to get her hair done. If she's gazing out the window, ask if she would like to go for a drive. Oftentimes, people with Alzheimer's aren't really interested in the destination – they just like to admire the passing scenery.

Take time to smell the roses. Sometimes smells evoke memories. Cut open a fresh lemon and hold it under your parent's nose and tell her stories about when you were a child and set up a sidewalk lemonade stand. Thank her for helping you make the lemonade.

Listen within your mind as you think of other smells that you and your parent experienced together, and what memories their aromas evoke. Did you walk through pine forests together? Did you go apple picking in the fall? Did she love the fragrance of plumeria leis from Hawaii or the night-blooming jasmine that grew outside her window?

Were there certain foods she cooked with that would evoke pleasant memories of shared times? Chop up some chilies and cilantro for her to smell and laugh about when the salsa was too spicy. Give her a small piece of chocolate to smell and then let her eat it and tell her how you loved to bake chocolate chip cookies with her.

What was your parent's favorite food? When Mom was near the end, we wanted her to experience her favorite flavor of ice cream again. Not expecting something special, she obediently opened her mouth to be fed, and the look of wonder on her smiling face as she tasted the chocolate ice cream was priceless.

Nothing you can think of is too silly. Don't second guess yourself by saying "Oh, he'd never remember that." There's a reason your thoughts are leading you to these ideas. Act on them, and see what fun you're still able to share together. Take some time now and then to just be still and listen, and you'll be amazed at the ideas you come up with that can make such an improvement in your interactions with your loved one.

Especially pay attention when your intuition tells you to ask for or give forgiveness. I got a very strong internal message that my mom did not want to pass on until she knew that her number two daughter had forgiven her for the turbulent teenage years of rebellion.

When I told my sister Genevieve, she was at first resistant to the idea. After a little thought though, she agreed, and phrased it so eloquently, saying, "Sherry has the impression that you want me to forgive you. I do forgive you, but there is really nothing to forgive. You always did what you felt was right and acted in the best interests of your children."

We decided it must have been what Mom wanted to hear. She became very alert, her whole countenance positively glowing with gratitude, as she gazed directly into my sister's eyes with love, blessing her with a big smile.

If your intuition is telling you to say or do something, you will feel better if you follow its advice. Before my dad passed away, I finally apologized for an incident that I had been beating myself up over for years because of my selfish and inconsiderate behavior. You know what happened when I asked for his forgiveness? He didn't even remember the incident! All these years I spent regretting my actions and longing for his forgiveness and he had forgiven me so long ago that he didn't even remember it.

Sometimes asking for forgiveness is more about fulfilling *your* needs than it is about the feelings of the person you felt you wronged.

If you feel you need to forgive your parent for any reason from the past, or for which you want to ask forgiveness, do it. Merely acting on it will set you free. You may even have a good laugh if she no longer remembers the incident. In going through this process, you realize that there's no point in holding on to resentment toward your parent for a past action when she no longer can remember or take responsibility for it.

It is a very healing realization.

Chapter 19
Love Endures with Quality Time

*"Whosoever loves much performs much,
and can accomplish much,
and what is done in love is done well."*
– Vincent Van Gogh

I remember when Mom could still talk and was so scared when we made a trip to the dentist. She sat in the dental chair and said to me, *"You're* the mommy now. *I'm* the baby." She wanted to be sure I knew that she trusted me to handle whatever situations she could no longer manage alone.

"Yes," I smiled. "I'm the mommy, and *you're* the baby now. That's okay. I like being your mommy, too."

It *was* a blessing to still have my mom with me. She was not the same, but she was still my mom, and the loving bond we shared had endured and strengthened over the years. Even through the pain and tears, we grew and evolved, and bonded ever more closely. Our love continued to grow and comfort us, a cushion that pushed back the reality as other outsiders would see it, and wrapped us in a special glow of togetherness, sharing a world so very different from the one we shared before, but still precious nonetheless.

I was grateful for the wonder of this experience. We had survived the rage and anger as well as the fear and despair, to find the love that was always there. Through all the years of my life, my mother's love for me had always been steadfast. It was good to find that my love for her was unfaltering as well.

I knew the day might come when we no longer had even the reality we knew now, but one thing I had learned. My mommy taught it to me, so indelibly that I would always remember her most significant lesson and legacy to me. **Love endures**.

Even so, as time went on, it got harder to visit. If Mom had a particularly good day the last time I visited, I wanted to hold onto that and savor the memory for awhile.

If she had a particularly bad day, it frightened me to think of what it would be like the next time I visited. And yet, each time I did go to see her, I felt uplifted by the experience. Yes, it was one of the hardest things I'd ever had to do, but at the same time, it was one of the most rewarding. For each time I felt that we connected with one another, on some level, and I came away knowing that I was loved, and knowing that she felt my love for her as well.

When I first arrived, she was usually looking off into space, seemingly unaware of her surroundings. But when I knelt down in front of her to put my face at her level, right in front of hers, and called, "Hi, Mom," she turned toward me and what I knew was a smile lit up her eyes, even if it was brief and fleeting. She was happy to know I was there and that I cared. After 15 years, how little it took to make us both happy.

Now that she could no longer walk or even stand on her own, I was content to be in her loving presence, and to shower my love onto her in return. The fat she carried was melting off her body and this once 200 pound woman now looked frail. I took my little ten pound Maltese doggie to visit her and sit on her lap, but found that even his slight weight was too much for her to bear, and she was no longer able to pet him and feel his soft fur. Sometimes I found it easier to visit if someone would go with me, but it is not a duty to impose on your children or spouse if they don't want to go. Luckily I had a friend who took care of her own mother with dementia and she understood and was willing to go with me occasionally. When my sisters came to town, we always visited our mom together and it was like a little celebration. These times were always the easiest. They now knew what to expect and seemed happy to just be with her.

Other friends and relatives occasionally asked to visit, but these times could be trying and emotional, as they hadn't prepared themselves for what they would encounter. After all, your loved one is just a shadow of their previous self.

So try not to use your children or spouse for support. They tend to be less help than you might think, and there's no point in making them resentful of you "dragging them along," when it's your own responsibility. Because they aren't familiar with how to connect to your loved one, they're uncomfortable, and it may not be worth the effort. When you go alone, you can stay as long as you want. I find even fifteen minutes is enough to let my mom know I care, feel a sense of peace and let tears flow if it feels right, and to smile through them as well, feeling the emotion.

It was a poignant time in our lives, so much like it must have been when I was a baby and we had no words to communicate with then either. So we did so by a touch, a look, a communion of souls. I was a fussy baby and cried a lot, so Mom carried me around propped on her hip, the constant warmth and reassurance of her body communicating itself to me.

How blessed we were now that I didn't have the daily responsibility of taking care of her every need, because I therefore spent only "quality time" with her, seeking to touch her within her recesses, to reach the depth of the person I knew as "Mother."

Usually, when I visited and I knelt by her side to place my face in front of hers, I also kissed her. Sometimes I played the game we played when I was a child, kissing first her forehead, then one cheek and then the other so, as my daddy used to say, "she won't fall over."

Sometimes we would "Eskimo kiss" by rubbing our noses together, and she seemed to enjoy this. Usually I held her hands and brought them to my lips for a kiss. One time I held her hands and must have forgotten the kiss, for she miraculously brought my hand to her lips and kissed it! What an incredible blessing.

How sweet is your mother's kiss. It was gifts like these that eased, that kept me honoring my mother by continuing to visit and shower my love upon her. For that is something no one can do just like you, the one she carried within her body for nine long months, creating a bond that remains, even now.

So continue to visit your parent and take what gifts she may be able to give. Even if you aren't sure at times if she knows you are there, your presence and your love reaches her on some level that we may not see or even be aware of. Try not to pressure yourself to go so often that you're resentful of the time you spend. Instead, space your visits every couple of weeks or so to give you time to compose yourself. Then when you are in her presence you can focus all of your attention and love on her, instead of concentrating on yourself and what you are feeling.

Remember that even though you may not want to go and face the reality of it all, when you are there something miraculous could happen. The veil over her eyes may rise and she may turn to you with such clarity that you *know* she knows you. How would you ever want to miss that? For if you are not there, the miracles can never happen to you or to her. So persevere, and count the blessings you have, for even though they may be fewer than you want, they are still there to be found if you only stay open and receptive.

Chapter 20
Keeper of Memories

"A hero is an ordinary individual who finds
the strength to persevere and endure
in spite of overwhelming obstacles."
- Christopher Reeve

I was now the keeper of the memories. I made journals and memory books for my mom, with photos and comments on important events and precious memories so we had a visual reminder. Sometimes Mom and I went through the books and I elaborated on all the fun we had at the occasions pictured. It was a positive way of coping with what was happening with the progression of my mom's disease. I highly suggest it. And it helps you hold the fear at bay – the lurking fear that perhaps you, too, will have memory problems in your old age.

You have plenty of time after your loved one is first diagnosed to take lots of pictures and videos. Think how wonderful your memories will be as you look back, as well as the fun to show your parent the story of her life. Interview relatives and friends, and get them to tell their stories on camera. My mom's best friend loves to tell the story of how Mom donated the baby carriage to the nursery school garage sale and then had to buy it back when she learned she was unexpectedly pregnant with me.

We watched videos from years ago when Mom could still swim in the pool. One favorite video featured one of many mock battles with the Styrofoam fun noodles, between my mom, my son and me, swinging the limp noodles like swords. I did the running commentary like a sportscaster: "...And Dan has the lead in fierce combat...now Grandma moves in to parry his thrusts...and round the pool they go, as this battle slips into overtime..." You get the idea.

Many people have a Thanksgiving tradition in which each person sitting at the table expresses why they are grateful. We videotaped our family tradition each Thanksgiving with family members reading funny jokes and stories we had collected during the year for this purpose. This way we could laugh again at the jokes when we watched the video, as it captured the sound of everyone's laughter and their appearance while they were all smiling and clearly having a good time.

My mom's favorite holiday was Halloween, and she always loved to dress up for it. We have a darling video of her wearing her witch costume, stirring the cauldron. When I asked her what she had in the pot, she had difficulty finding the words to answer, so I suggested she use the soup ladle to show us. I paused the recording, put a fake eyeball in the ladle she held up, and then restarted the filming. It turned out great!

The memory scrapbook I made for Mom is now a priceless family heirloom. You can take classes at a craft store that show you how to use acid-free paper, pens and stickers to create archival-quality albums that will preserve the pictures from fading over the years. Your loved ones will know how much you care when you spend the time and energy to create such a lasting legacy, one that can be handed down through the generations. Several Web sites enable you to scan your photos, add copy and publish a finished book.

I started by finding pictures of Mom's parents, the sepia tones and old-time fashions clearly showing the difference of the times. I found out all the stories I could about her growing up; how she met and married Daddy; the births of each child; and the homes they had. I included the best stories from each time period and found photos to match the stories. If your loved one travelled but you can't find a photo of the destinations, you can include a picture postcard. Since my father was an artist, I included some of his artwork, such as my birth announcement cartoon and several of the zany Christmas cards we created as a family project every December.

Find the precious bits and pieces that tend to disappear over time and let them live on in the photo album, like the macaroni necklace Mom's daughter made for her or the popsicle stick jewelry box from the scout camping trip which she treasured. Many families save handprints of the kids when they were little, which would be perfect to include.

If your parents remodeled their home, include the before and after pictures. If they won an award, include the certificate. In one file I found all of my mother's letters of recommendations she had collected over the years from her employers. These were absolutely glowing tributes to her, so I included them in the back of the book.

As you clean out your parents' papers, look for precious finds such as the autobiography my father wrote. Granted it was in tiny, barely legible handwriting on various scraps of paper, but he told some great stories. I found a newspaper article my father clipped years ago about my grandfather and found out things I never knew about him. I also found a few pages of a "This is Your Life" script Dad used for a party for Mom – priceless memories that would have otherwise been lost.

Keep taking pictures as the years progress. Keep only the ones you like, where your loved one looks alert, and throw the rest away. I have pictures of us at church, pictures from our walks in the park, pictures sitting in the garden, pictures with the relatives when they came to visit. If I had stopped taking photos, I would have missed capturing lots of years and memories. At the times I took the pictures, I really wasn't sure if I would want them. People have a tendency to think their loved one doesn't look good anymore. Yet when you see the photos after time has passed, it can be a comfort to remember all that you were able to share together.

As your parent loses his memories, you can be the one who keeps them as the treasures they are. You don't have to be artistic to create this. Just gather the photos and you'll be surprised how easily it comes together. Your parent will be pleased and impressed that you feel his life was important enough to chronicle. You can take comfort knowing that once your parent is gone, his stories will be remembered by the rest of the family, and newly born members will have a sense of their ancestors by what you memorialize in the book.

If your parent has grandchildren, it's nice to show pictures of them together from birth through their growing older together. You might consider having a section dedicated to each grandchild. Then when the grandchildren come to visit, they're more apt to sit with their grandparent to review "their" section of the book. Include stories from their perspective and in their words if you like. For example, could their grandparent magically pull a quarter out of his ear?

Ask the grandchildren what they liked to do or what

was special when they visited Grandma's house. Record their answers and include them in the book. Did they like to color pictures together? Did they find a special item or plaything at Grandma's that could be found nowhere else? My aunt had a special ceramic chicken that magically laid, not an egg, but a shiny coin for me, before I left her house. My son said Grandma always fixed him eggs and they always tasted better at her house.

When I decided to make a film for Mom's memorial, I used the scrapbook as a basis for it. I scanned the photos into the computer and recorded my voice telling each story. Many computer programs show you step by step how to produce a show and burn it to a disc. I used "HP (Hewlett Packard) Image Zone" and it included many different ways to transition to the next photo, such as various wipes and fades, making it a very professional-looking, finished product.

This is a labor of love and takes time to research. You may want to include quotes from friends and loved ones. You may want to start with a family photograph of the ancestors and tell when they arrived in the country. Include family stories. Our favorite one tells of Grandma making wine in the bathtub during Prohibition days. You can use the important formal pictures, such as graduation and wedding photos, as well as snapshots of your loved ones having fun with other family members.

Whatever physical form the memories take, it's a real treasure to keep and a legacy to share with your family.

Chapter 21
Be There for the Special Moments

"Beautiful young people are accidents of nature,
but beautiful old people are works of art."
–Eleanor Roosevelt

While the state-of the-art Alzheimer's Special Care Unit was truly wonderful when we moved Mom in, over time we noticed more and more changes to it. First, the staff started charging extra for dry cleaning every month and I had to remind them that I would not pay because my mother no longer owned any garments that needed dry cleaning. Then they sent a letter asking each resident to pay $50 for lunch when they took them out on drives. I said no, because I was already paying lots of money for her food that was included at the facility and at this point my mother could barely eat *any* food, let alone $50 worth at one sitting.

These were little annoyances, but when I found the wonderful people who had been caring for Mom had been laid off and replaced with what could be termed "far less savory" people, I began to be concerned. Once when I came to pick up Mom, it was clear to my nose that her diaper needed changing. When I asked for this service, I was appalled to learn that a male, rather than a female, was assigned to change her diapers. When I clearly told the new administrator that this was unacceptable, she said it was common practice unless it was otherwise noted on the patient's chart. My response was, "How would I have known that I had to *request* a female attendant to change my mother's diapers?"

The final straw came one day when I picked up Mom. She could barely walk as she hobbled toward me. She wasn't wearing the lovely, thin socks I had given her (one of many pairs labeled with her name), but had been dressed in someone else's thick, bulky socks, which caused her great difficulty because her shoes didn't fit over them properly. When I took off her shoes and socks, I noticed a horrible blister this had caused on her heel and it was clear her feet had not been properly dried as they were wet between her toes.

So, although the place you choose for your loved one may be wonderful at the time you move in, you need to constantly monitor the situation to be sure it remains that way. Luckily for us, Mom grew out of her aggressive stage after about a year's time, as her ability to express anger diminished, and we moved her back to Mary's care. Mary owned more than one board and care home and we settled Mom into a different home far away from Emma.

My mother had been very specific that she wanted "no heroic means" used to keep her alive. She had discussed this with me and signed the official "Do Not Resuscitate" (DNR) form, which made it much easier on me. A newer and nicer name for this is "AND" which means "Allow Natural Death." If this is the way your loved one feels about the issue, have them sign the form, as it will give you a measure of peace around your decisions. (These and other forms are discussed in detail in Chapter 3.)

Mom instructed me that when the time came and there was no hope of getting better, that she wanted me to let her go naturally. She specifically wrote down, "No feeding tube, no intravenous, no ventilator or respirator."

One thing we had not thought to specify was antibiotics. This turned out to be a point of conflict. For my mom, as is frequently the case in Alzheimer's patients near the end, her swallowing mechanism began to fail. When this happens, food and liquid can go down into the lungs instead of the stomach, and pneumonia often results. Pneumonia can be treated with antibiotics, so the decision to be made was: Would Mom want antibiotics even though it could prolong her life or would Mom prefer that nature take its course and just go?

Her 200 pound body had shrunk to less than 150 pounds in the preceding weeks. Her lack of circulation had left patches of blackened gangrenous skin on her feet, and she developed bedsores which would not heal. I knew she was ready to give up the fight under these conditions. Mary, the owner of the board and care home, did not feel it was morally right for her to keep Mom unless she gave her antibiotics, which would ease Mom's difficulties with her cough and fever from the pneumonia. She felt they did not fall under the DNR heading of "heroic measures," but they would be able to make Mom more comfortable.

Therefore, if I chose not to give Mom antibiotics, I would have to move her to a nursing home. I didn't want to make my mom go through the trauma of another move, new surroundings and new caregivers.

When I saw how Mom's body was giving up the fight, I called my sisters and explained the situation. We would have to move Mom to a nursing home in order to let her pass on.

Both sisters strongly felt that Mom couldn't have meant to *not* give her antibiotics since they weren't considered a "heroic" measure, like hooking her up to machines to keep her alive. At first I agreed, and we gave Mom the antibiotics. Then it became apparent once Mom took the medication and got well, that the cycle of pneumonia started all over again in another several days. I was very troubled by this development, and the hospice nurse said this pattern would keep repeating.

I was torn by my desire to have Mom pass away in the same comfortable surroundings of the home she had been living in for the past few years now, surrounded by her loving caretakers who bestowed hugs and kisses and affection on her throughout each day. I was horrified that I now had to face a move to one of "those" places where, to my eyes, all the old people who aren't your mom look crazy, and the people on staff are unfamiliar with you and your mom and don't seem as caring, and it oftentimes smells bad. I clearly didn't want to see her in unpleasant surroundings, as it's hard enough seeing her in the beautiful place where she's living.

The hospice doctor was quite unequivocal and helped me see the situation with great clarity. When he picked up Mom's medical chart, he looked at the "Do Not Resuscitate" form and asked, "Did your mother speak with you about her wishes on this?"

I said, "Yes, she was very clear that I was not to use artificial means to prolong her life."

He harshly said, "Then why are you giving her antibiotics?"

I explained Mary's viewpoint – that she morally had to administer them to keep Mom more comfortable and in less pain. I told him my sisters' viewpoint – that God would take her when He was ready, even if she were on antibiotics.

The doctor looked me in the eye and firmly said, "There is *no question* that you are prolonging her life with antibiotics. You are *NOT* doing what your mother asked you to do." At this time, I looked at my mom's face, and I swear she was giving me a really dirty look that echoed what the doctor said.

While most people would have found the doctor brutally blunt, it was what I needed to hear. He was right. While Mom had not specifically addressed the use of antibiotics, she had been very clear – do not prolong my life. Let me go. At that moment, I knew the doctor's words to be the truth. I had absolute clarity that this was what Mom's and my talks had been about, this was what Mom wanted now and this was the correct course to take. If she could talk to me now, she would tell me not to prolong her agonies. She had suffered enough. I beg you to have this talk with your loved ones while they are of sound mind in order to clarify their desires and make your job easier to accept and perform.

I asked Mary if, given the circumstances that I would be moving Mom in a few days, she would be willing to keep her without antibiotics until the nursing home could take her. She agreed, and explained that she was not without feelings, and that was why she had asked me to move Mom. Mary and her family had cared for Mom for so long and at such an intimate level that she felt Mom was part of her family. She was hoping Mom would pass away quietly in her sleep (didn't we all) but the doctor said if we kept giving her antibiotics, Mom could hang on for even several more months. That was exactly what Mom had warned me against and so my path was crystal clear.

Members of your family who don't live nearby and haven't watched the transition may be reluctant to accept that their parent is dying. You, who have been going through the reality of life and death on a daily basis, may need to help them understand the changes and the condition of your loved one. You may need to be the one to impress upon them that if they want to say goodbye in person, now is the time to come. Even then, it may take time and more than one conversation for it all to sink in.

That's not to say that it's easy for you to be the one to let them know. Or easy on you if they decide not to come. You may find it difficult to understand why you have to be the one to shoulder not only the realities of caring for your loved one, but also taking on the load of letting siblings know and trying to make them understand the emotional, practical and physical realities of what's going on there with your parent.

You may be hoping that your siblings will come out at this critical moment to say goodbye and to support you. Realize that each of us has our own decisions to make for ourselves and some may find it more difficult than others. They are going through their own emotions of dealing with your loved one's condition, whether or not they have an accurate viewpoint or are capable of understanding. You can only tell them the prognosis. It's up to them to decide whether or not to come. You have no power to make them come, so release any concerns you may have about it.

I called my sisters more than once to tell them the time was near. It was a turbulent and difficult time. They said they had already said their goodbyes and resisted coming. Perhaps it was too difficult to face. Perhaps they didn't grasp the reality of it all.

Should you encounter a similar situation, I suggest composing a letter to your family members. I sent my sisters this frank letter explicitly detailing Mom's condition, that she had about one week left to live and asked them to please come help me.

Dear Sisters,

I have to admit, it would be so much easier on us to let Mom pass away at Mary's. However, Mom was very clear that we were not to use any means to prolong her life. Her clear intention was that we are to release her and let her go. I do so hope, as we all do, that God allows her to die soon and at Mary's. It's difficult to see Mom in her deteriorated state and I think if you were here and saw what she is going through, it may change your mind about coming.

Do I want to move her to a nursing home? No. Do I want her to pass on as quickly and easily as possible? We all do. So while I have been sparing you the ugly graphic details of Mom's current condition, I need to share them with you now.

Mom has shrunk from 200 pounds to about 150 or less, which is extremely frail and bony for her. Patches of gangrene infect her feet like Daddy's before he died. She has broken off her teeth by grinding them (teeth grinding is a symptom of pain.) Open-wound bedsores cover the crack of her behind that are about the size of her open hand-span. She has almost totally lost the ability to swallow food, so she is not getting nourishment, and will be starving. Because of her bedsores, she can no longer sit up, can only lie on her side, and needs to be turned every two hours. Changing her diapers is a long, involved and painful process to her, and it must be done regularly or the bedsores will get worse.

As you know, Mom contracted pneumonia ten days ago and is now going through her second bout, both with antibiotics. As we discussed, Mom wanted no part of extending

167

her life. It's in her best interest to not keep giving her antibiotics, because as the hospice nurse said, the cycle of catching pneumonia, recovering and catching it again will just keep repeating. They say that pneumonia is a friend to the old and ailing because it allows them to pass on.

We all hope Mom transitions soon at Mary's. If she does not, and gets pneumonia again, we need to transfer her to the nursing home in order to let her die. Mary will not take care of her if we don't give her antibiotics.

The hospice nurse says that with pneumonia, Mom will pass in a week. Without it, she may take a month. This is not the kind of life that anyone would want to prolong, especially for another whole month. I'm letting you know these blunt facts because if Mom gets pneumonia again, we will need to move her so that we can allow her to go.

I would like you to be here to help me through this. I understand you may not feel you need to be here to say goodbye for yourself, but this is the end of a 16 year journey for me of intense care, of my life being impacted weekly and oftentimes daily by Mom, and I, as your sister, am asking for your help and support.

I don't want to go through this alone if I don't have to. If you could both come out, we could then transfer Mom to the nursing home and the three of us can be there to help Mom release and let go. Please contemplate this and let me know.

Let us all pray that Mom transitions soon so that we don't need to face anything else.

If she does not, I think it is only kind to move her so she can pass on, without the artificial aid of antibiotics prolonging her suffering.

My sisters agreed to come.

At some level, you need to understand how difficult it is for family members that have stayed away. Perhaps they want to preserve the last memories they have of their parent, when she wasn't so ill. You need to have charity in your heart for the shock it will be to them. Perhaps that's why, when you first ask them to come, they resist so strongly – they don't want it to be true and they don't want to see their parent like this.

One day it was apparent Mom's bodily functions were all starting to fail at once. When I entered her room and saw her I asked, "Are you ready to hang it up and go see Daddy in heaven?"

She clearly looked at me and moved her head ever so slightly up and down to nod a most definite "Yes." Moments like this let me know it was time. I told her she had put up a good fight, and if she was ready to go, that would be okay with me.

While Mom and I waited for her other daughters to arrive, I was blessed every day. Mom would be sleeping or staring vacantly when I arrived at her bedside, but once she became aware that I was there, she had a clarity that was exceptional for her advanced stage of Alzheimer's.

I got up close to her face, so it was easy for her to focus on me, and told her she was the best mommy in the world – that I was her baby, and she was my baby now. I thanked her for giving me life, and then for all the love and care she gave to me throughout the half a century we were together. I would play "Nosie, Nosie" with her, rubbing our noses together. Her nose would be cold due to poor circulation, and I would remind her that both she and puppy dogs had cold noses, just as we played when I was young.

On a good day, when her eyes seemed bright and clear,

she not only seemed to recognize me, but we spoke volumes to one another through our eyes meeting in simple silence.

We were closer than ever, treasuring our precious shared moments. I took my choir hymnal one day and went through it from cover to cover, singing all of the tunes we had heard in church, but most of all, the Christmas carols. After a long while, I asked her, "Are you tired of my singing?"

She actually moved her head to indicate no while a sound of negativity pushed passed her lips. Amazed, I asked, "Would you like me to sing more?"

She responded by smiling, almost imperceptibly nodding yes. My heart soared, and we enjoyed all the carols again. I wanted so much for my sisters to have that blessed time of communion with my mother, like I had.

The day after Mom and I had our "song fest," my eldest sister arrived. Mom was not as alert as the day before, but when Stephanie came in and I told Mom her number one daughter had arrived, she opened her eyes and a clear smile of recognition brightened her entire countenance.

The two of them had a wonderful visit, with my Mom pouring all of her love out to my sister through her eyes, and my sister drinking it all in and returning her love. It was so healing and perfect.

The very next day, I announced to Mom that her number two daughter had arrived. Although Mom was a little frailer, the same beautiful experience recurred. She awakened to see Genevieve and her eyes cleared and a big smile of recognition spread across her face. She was so incredibly happy that both my sisters had come, and she showered all of us with her love.

We sat at her bedside and told her all the things we

wanted her to know in our mind-to-mind communication. This was what I had hoped for and wanted – for my sisters to experience the beauty of what I had with Mom. For one last time to have that total acceptance of our mother's love shining out on them. How perfect it was.

Chapter 22
Forewarned is Forearmed

"Whoever doesn't know it must learn
and find by experience that
a quiet conscience makes one strong."
– Anne Frank

We were ready now. After experiencing the great grace our mother poured forth...and after she showered us with an all knowing, profound love that we all shared during those perfect moments, my sisters and I prepared for the logistics of the next day. As recommended by the medical team, we moved Mom to the nursing home. When we first arrived, the doctor was so very kind and accommodating, and said she would respect our wishes for no artificial means to prolong Mom's life.

The doctor also said they would not disturb Mom while she was sleeping. Yet every fifteen minutes for two hours they came in to try and take her vital signs, while my eldest sister asked them to come back when Mom was awake. The staff finally insisted and we had to confront the doctor who begrudgingly backed down.

Next, I had to sign the admission papers to the nursing home. If you have insurance, this can be very difficult, as I found out. Although a social worker had been assigned to me to presumably help us, she was not forthcoming with all the details. She had said she would help me apply for state aid for nursing home care (Medi-Cal) before we had to place Mom in the nursing facility. She said that our preferred provider organization (PPO) would cover only *one week*, and the remainder would be our responsibility. Since Mom didn't have much money left after 16 years of care, I was most concerned about qualifying for aid, and was panicked about having to sign anything that said I would be responsible.

Having been my mom's trustee for so many years, I had been trained to read everything I signed, even if it consisted of pages and pages of single-spaced typing. Much to the nursing home staff's annoyance, I read it all. What concerned me the most was a little phrase hidden in pages of legalese that said by admitting my mom under hospice, I was giving up her rights to Medicare. I needed clarification on this, as it didn't sound right to me, and was not what I had understood from the social worker. In addition, the papers said I would be responsible for all supplies and I knew that could add incredible expenses.

If I had to sign something in writing, I wanted to know exactly what Mom's insurance was covering in writing. I refused to sign the admittance papers and put in an urgent call to the social worker, who did not call me back. You cannot believe the intense pressure they brought to bear on me to sign the papers, hour after hour, with them repeatedly saying, "We can figure that all out later."

Beware – if you are upset and don't read the paperwork carefully, once you have signed it, you have no legal recourse. Three people were "ganging up on me" – the admittance clerk, her supervisor and the department head – all trying to convince me to sign the forms, whether I understood them or not, because "they were just there to help Mom."

We were *all* getting upset. When Mom left her room at the board and care home to come here, she was peaceful. Now she had wrinkles on her forehead. We were frustrated with the

174

admissions and the staff, and everything was going downhill fast.

While the staff said they would take every measure to comfort Mom, we didn't understand what their concept of "comfort" measures included. The proverbial "straw that broke the camel's back" for us was when they decided – for Mom's "comfort" – to suspend her in a sling from the ceiling so she would put less pressure on her bedsores. Mom was already on the inflatable mattress that hospice provided for transporting her to the nursing home, as it was least painful to simply lift the mattress onto the hospital gurney rather than touch Mom to move her. Does it make sense that a woman who wanted to die naturally and peacefully should be suspended from the ceiling in a sling? We didn't think so. Especially since she was going to pass on probably very quickly, regardless of her bedsores, due to her pneumonia.

Now here's the really interesting part. Although our hospice nurse and social worker had originally said they expected my mom would only live one week once she was moved to the nursing home, the doctor there said Mom was stable, her lungs didn't sound like she had pneumonia after all, and she might live several more months. It's possible that the antibiotics cleared the pneumonia, but what about their insistence that she would just contract it again?

My sisters and I had based moving our mom to the nursing home on Mary saying she could not forgo giving Mom antibiotics and she didn't want to have to watch her die. Also, because we had thought – based on what the medical experts told us – it would only be about a week before Mom passed on. We knew the insurance paid for a week. It may be uncharitable to think it, but it felt like the nursing home staff just wanted to get us into the nursing home and then collect money once Mom did *not* pass away. I know all of this is terrible to think about, but this is what happened to us. Forewarned is forearmed.

We pleaded with the nursing home staff to return Mom to her board and care home. After four and a half hours they finally gave up trying to keep her at the nursing home against our wishes, and let us take her back (although we of course had to pay for the hospital gurney ride back). When Mom saw she was once again back in her beautiful room with the smiling faces of her usual caregivers, she broke into a weak but heartfelt smile and we all felt we had done the right thing to bring her back. I should mention that Mary had now accepted my decision to let Mom pass on, and was willing to keep her without administering any additional antibiotics.

Now we embarked on the fight with our insurance provider to state the specific coverage Mom had in writing. At this point, I talked to four different representatives, and each one told me a different story, varying from five days coverage to 90 days – a difference of many thousands of dollars.

I told our medical provider and their hospice representatives in no uncertain terms that I thought they were there to help me, and yet they had only caused my family and me extreme stress and grief. Finally, they confessed that if Mom were to be admitted to the nursing home under the hospice program, the insurance only covered five days for respite care or seven days for General In Patient (GIP).

However, if I discharged Mom off of hospice, she could be admitted to the nursing home under the "Skilled Care Benefit." Under this long term benefit, the insurance would pay until her bedsores healed.

Since her bedsores were at Stage Three (Stage Four is where the wound goes down to the bone), it didn't seem likely that they would be healed before she passed on, or at least not for a good long while.

In my complaint to the hospice director, I mentioned that the social worker had not assisted me in applying for state aid and I did not find out until after moving Mom to the nursing home that the application takes 45 days after it's submitted to be approved. Since we started talking to hospice, we had already wasted ten days. Also, they don't tell you unless you specifically ask, but you are much more likely to get approval if the nursing home submits the paperwork, rather than you submitting it directly.

In California, there are specific rules for qualifying for state aid. In this instance, if we had Mom in a hospital for three days and nights and then transferred her to the nursing home, she was virtually assured of coverage. If, however, we took her to the nursing home without a three day hospital stay (which, in our ignorance, is what we did), she would not qualify for coverage.

Although this example of our experience may be painful to read, please benefit from what we went through. Ask your insurance provider for their specific coverage for your specific case BEFORE you get to the nursing home. Get the application for government assistance online, fill it out and take it to the nursing home BEFORE you have to admit your loved one and ask them if they will submit on your loved one's behalf. They can only say no; they may say yes, and you will at least get them to submit it on the very first day of your loved one's stay.

Also, I didn't realize that there was a vast difference

between different hospice providers. I had been dealing with the hospice provided by our medical plan. However conscientious they try to be, it appears to me that there may be a conflict of interest when the people advising you to put your loved one in a nursing home know their employer will save thousands of dollars if they can get you to commit to circumstances that your medical coverage will not cover.

I was not aware of it at the time, but you have a choice of using any hospice you would like. You are not obligated to use the hospice program provided by your health care insurance. Based on my experiences, I would choose a hospice without a connection to the insurance provider. The incredibly loving, wonderful hospice experience (www.buenav istahospicecare.com) we later had with my husband's mother was far more supportive and caring than the experience I had with the medical insurance hospice.

Thankfully, my sisters were with me the whole time to help with their loving support.

Ah, if only that blessing of support could linger indefinitely. But sibling friction is something every family will experience in one way or another, to one degree or another, over different aspects of a journey such as this. Experts say no family escapes it. A parent going through Alzheimer's brings out raw emotions, old hurts (real or perceived), confusion and misunderstandings, regrets of things done or left undone, in all family members.

Each individual has their own understanding of the disease and concepts of how to cope with the demands it presents. Each family member has their own personality along with different styles and views on how various situations should be handled. Each sibling has a different relationship with their parent which can influence their perceptions. The stress level will be high if one feels very guilty, resentful, sad, frightened or overwhelmed. The emotional elements and family dynamics can cause great upheaval.

We sisters had some painful issues in the past over the fact that I was chosen as trustee and had control over Mom's funds. Hurt invaded, too, when I felt Stephanie and Genevieve did not come through on their pledges to help with caregiving. And there were times when my sisters clearly didn't trust me. We spent many years cautiously rebuilding our relationships and forgiving one another while on the roller coaster ride of Mom's Alzheimer's.

Inheritance is just one more aspect that can strain relationships, especially when participants have different viewpoints. Mom and Dad had bought four diamonds years ago, one for each of the three daughters and one for Mom's sister, Min. We decided that since we were all here together, and the inevitable end was near, we would distribute the diamonds now. My eldest sister was now caring for Aunt Min, who couldn't enjoy the diamond as she was now in the throes of Alzheimer's, and we all agreed Stephanie should get Min's diamond, too.

It was a blow to discover the diamonds were not in the safe as expected when we opened it. We all remembered the story differently as to who did what with them for storage. We said things that hurt, and we all parted horribly upset, without the diamonds. I had never expected this twist of fate to once more tear our affections for one another apart. It wasn't until a year later, as Stephanie and I talked, that we figured out our memories had played tricks on each of us. It turned out that, through actions on both our parts, the diamonds ended up tucked away in Mom's files in a large envelope and not in the safe at all. I quickly retrieved them, insured them and sent them off to my sisters.

It helps greatly in preventing tattered fabrics of family relationships if all involved work to openly communicate with each other. Try to see things from the others' points of view. Make the first goal be to make it work. Be strong and be polite.

And, as challenging as it may be, learn to let things go.

Chapter 23
Nursing Options

"Do or Do not. There is no <u>Try</u>."
– Yoda, Star Wars Master

As it turned out, the prognosis for "Mom's passing in a week's time" extended to over two years more. Obviously, giving her antibiotics was not the best choice, as it unquestionably lengthened the time Mom continued to be trapped in a body and mind that were no longer functioning. Once again we needed to find a way to care for Mom which would not be so expensive.

How can you put a value on caring for your loved one in a place other than an institutional nursing home? When Mom's money ran out, we had to choose to either put her in the care of the government or find a way to come up with the substantial amount of money needed for her to continue to live in the nicest home environment with a 24 hour a day caregiver who loved my mom. Is it worth mortgaging your house? Is it worth spending your retirement money? You have to be fair to your own family as well.

Each time I explored the nursing home option, I ran into road blocks. Because my mother had worked for the state government, she had their contracted medical plan instead of Medicare. In order to qualify for Medicare coverage, we would have to cancel her medical plan and, once cancelled, we could never get it back.

Mom's bedsores had gone from a Stage 4 (meaning the

flesh was open to the bone) to being healed by meticulous care, including the use of a catheter so she wouldn't be sitting in wet diapers. When Mom was on the medical provider's hospice plan, they provided an inflatable mattress to more evenly distribute her weight and her caregiver turned her every two hours. The reward was that Mom was no longer in pain, but the down side was that since her bedsores improved (something the medical plan said was virtually impossible) she no longer qualified to have the inflatable bed which had helped her heal.

The medical plan took the bed away and sent instead a worthless mattress cover. When Mom didn't expire after the allotted six month time span that hospice allows, the medical plan took her off hospice care, but for a while at least still sent a nurse to check on her periodically.

We had a "Catch-22" situation. While Mom had her severe bedsores, she could be admitted to the nursing home as needing "skilled care," a condition which we were told the medical plan would cover for one to two weeks and the nursing home would be willing to apply for Medicare while she was there.

Because her bedsores healed, however, she no longer "qualified" as needing "skilled care." Instead, it was considered "custodial" care. Therefore, the nursing home wouldn't take her unless she already had been *pre-approved* for Medicare coverage. Yet when I wanted to confirm that they would take her once she was approved, they said that their Medicare beds were already full and they wouldn't accept her.

So the legal counsel who said that the nursing home would apply for the Medicare coverage was not completely correct – not unless you could prove your patient needed "skilled care." The fact that our meticulously conscientious care had helped Mom heal was now what prevented her coverage. Did I want to trust the care of my loved one to a place who operated like this? No. Did I have another choice? I hoped so.

I started by searching the Internet and found the most helpful site for me was the official United States government site for Medicare (www.medicare.gov/NHcompare). It lists all facilities that are approved to care for those receiving government aid. Each of these facilities is required to have periodic reviews by government inspectors, and the website lists any treatment deficiencies that have been found. Some of these I considered to be minor, such as failing to "provide activities to meet the needs of each resident."

Some deficiencies listed, however, were alarming to me, such as the following:

"Inspectors determined that the nursing home failed to:
- Protect each resident from all abuse, physical punishment, and being separated from others.
- Keep each resident free from physical restraints, unless needed for medical treatment.
- 1) Make sure that residents who take drugs are not given too many doses or for too long; 2) make sure that the use of drugs is carefully watched; or 3) stop or change drugs that cause unwanted effects."

In addition, the site notes the national average amount of time spent daily with each patient (i.e. 1 hour, 12 minutes for nursing staff hours and 2 hours, 18 minutes for certified nursing assistant hours) and compares the amount of time each facility spends, so you can evaluate how the home measures up to national and state averages.

The Medicare site also lists 15 quality measures for each facility versus the national average. They include categories such as the percentage of residents who had pressure sores (bedsores), were physically restrained, and had a urinary tract infection. These categories reflect on the quality of care provided by the nursing home and are an indicator of whether or not you would find the facility's care acceptable.

I found that when I was in practical mode, focused on finding an answer to our situation, I could objectively analyze this data, as unpalatable as it was. However, when I visited my mom, when I looked at her sweet face and her expression seemed to indicate pain or fear, my natural inclination was to reassure her that, although her life was difficult now, I was doing everything possible to make it as pleasant as possible. How can you say "I wish I could make everything better" and not do whatever it takes to keep her in a loving home instead of giving her over to institutional care?

Today as I sang to her one of her favorite songs, "Count Your Blessings," at least we had some to count. We counted our love for each other, and my mom's caretakers and her lovely surroundings at the board and care home. She had soft classical music playing in her private room instead of two noisy roommates in hospital beds next to her and all the clamor of activity in the halls of a nursing home. It was very peaceful here and she had a window to look outside. How much easier it was to visit her in such surroundings.

Psychologists say that when confronted with a difficult decision, people often concentrate on an either/or choice, rather than looking at all possible options. Dr. Laura Schlessinger said oftentimes on her radio program that a mother sometimes has to stand her ground and make up her mind that she's going to stay home to take care of her child (instead of working) no matter what budgeting is needed to make it happen. Yoda, the diminutive sage from the Star Wars series, says *"Do or Do not; there is no 'Try"* meaning that once you make up your mind not to just "try," but to "do" whatever it takes, you will find a way.

I knew in my heart that the perfect spot for my mother existed at a price we could figure out how to manage. For us, the residential care option provided the best quality – we just needed to find one that was less expensive now. I envisioned Mom sharing a cheerful room in a board and care home located closer to me, where there would be two full-time caregivers living at the house to take care of the six residents.

Right away I found the perfect spot that I had visualized. After meeting the caregivers and seeing what would be Mom's room, I knew immediately that this was the best place for us. However, the price they quoted was beyond our means, so they showed me other homes they managed which were less expensive. Luckily, the owner could tell I really wanted the "perfect spot" we had seen earlier, and I was thrilled that she was willing to negotiate and come down on the cost so we could afford it.

It was time to evaluate the few assets we had left, such as the silver saved in case of another depression, and the gold watches and jewelry. I took them all to an appraiser and was pleased to find out that the price of silver and gold was up and we could actually get a substantial amount of cash for our valuables. Of course, we wouldn't part with my mother's wedding ring or the few pieces of jewelry which we siblings were attached to on a sentimental level. However, in the safe I found gold watches and old coins that none of us had ever seen. In the hopes that one of these old coins would be rare and worth cash, I took everything to be evaluated and then decided what we could part with to help Mom's situation.

I thought of one option which I hoped might keep some level of peace in the family: to offer that family members could purchase whichever items they wanted at the same price I could receive for them, and see if they felt strongly enough to purchase the item at the bargain price. If they weren't interested, I concluded that the item was not of significant enough value to them, and traded it for cash to use toward Mom's care.

Chapter 24
Coping with Medical Providers

"If you run into a wall,
don't turn around and give up.
Figure out how to climb it,
go through it or work around it."
– Michael Jordan

If you belong to a large health care provider, there is both good news and bad news. When you have a primary care physician you like, the system works very well. You can develop a relationship with him or her, and they will be instrumental in seeing that your loved one receives the care she needs and deserves. They can also be helpful to *you*, providing you with valuable information, counseling sessions, and assigning a social worker who can advise you on many of the issues you're facing.

Be advised, however, that if your relationship with your doctor lapses, or you're assigned to a new doctor, you can be facing the problem of no one knowing or caring who you are. When we were seeing Mom's physician regularly, he was a great resource. But once Mom was bedridden and unable to go in to see the doctor, he forgot who she was, and each time I called I was told that he would not write any prescriptions for her because "he had never seen her."

Although I explained that we had been in to see him many times, they no longer had a record of Mom in the computer because it had been a lapse of four years since her last visit. They had changed computer systems four years ago, and anyone who had not been in to see a doctor since then was listed in the computer with their name and medical record number and the note: "no information."

I explained that if the doctor looked in her chart, he would see that we had been there numerous times and had in fact been seeing him for years, and I had even brought in Mom's sister to see him – he was the one who diagnosed Aunt Min with Alzheimer's. His assistant, who I was told I had to deal with because I couldn't talk with the doctor (because he had no record of Mom being his patient), even claimed, "He's a very young doctor, I don't think you have the right person."

What you may not realize is that doctors with these large health care providers don't actually have the charts of their patients. They have to order the chart to be sent to them, and if they don't have a record in the computer that your loved one has been in to see them, she is literally thought of as not being their patient and they will not even agree to order the chart.

Furthermore, because he had no record of Mom being his patient, he would not agree to even talk with me, so I had no way of reminding him who we were and what he'd done for us, such as the time he cut a large cyst out of her back and we kept her from getting upset by giving her a lollypop. I thought we had a great relationship and we did – the problem was that after four years of other patients, he didn't remember us.

Therefore, it's wise to always keep in touch with your primary care physician. I recommend you ask your health care provider to do a checkup once a year. This will keep their medical file updated on how your loved one is progressing, including significant details such as "she has lost weight, she now eats only pureed foods," etc.

At this time the Medicare rules stated that without the doctor's written request, one could not receive *any* medication or services such as Home Health Care or Hospice. After much criticism over this policy, Medicare recently relaxed the rules somewhat for hospice patient medications. (AARP Bulletin, September 2014).

By Mom's falling fall off the computer screen through lack of contact, we found ourselves in a "no-man's land," becoming a bother they hope will go away if they just keep repeating that they have no record of us.

If this has happened to you, there is still hope. Don't frustrate yourself by trying to fix the problem over the phone, for then you're a faceless voice which is easy to ignore. You must go in person, and hopefully find someone who has compassion and is willing to help you. Realize going in that this is oftentimes not going to be the first person you talk to about your predicament. Exercise patience, but be firm in your resolve so they know you are not going to go away, and that sooner or later something will have to be done for you.

If you have a social worker assigned to your case, that person is a good place to start. If not, start at Member Services. If you can bring another person with you, such as another family member, it strengthens your case measurably, as well as helps support you in your quest. Such was the case when I walked into the doctor's office, with my sister Genevieve, who happened to be in town at the time.

Realize that you never know where your help is going to come from, so be especially kind to everyone you meet, always make eye contact, ask their name and introduce yourself. We did this with the woman who was working the front desk at Member Services. I glanced at the name plate on the desk and asked if she were that person. As it turned out, she was not and was substituting that day. I asked her name, introduced myself, made eye contact and calmly explained our predicament. She suggested that we get a Home Health Care evaluation of Mom, and I explained that was exactly what I wanted, and was how we had taken care of the problem one previous time, when Mom was too weak to be transported in to see the doctor. She paged the social worker while I sat patiently in the lobby, well within her line of sight. When the social worker didn't answer her personal pager, she paged her over the intercom, while I expressed my gratitude.

Unfortunately, when the social worker finally arrived, she had the mindset of many who work in the system – that "the rules are the rules." And the rules say they cannot prescribe medication of any kind without the doctor seeing the patient. The doctor will not see the patient anywhere but the clinic. When I explained that my mother was in such a fragile state of health that her caregiver advised it could literally kill Mom to transport her to the clinic, she still insisted it was the only way.

I said it didn't seem right to take a chance of killing my mother just to get her medication such as over-the-counter Tylenol® to alleviate her pain. I asked what they would do if it were *their* mother and everyone I dealt with categorically stated that they would still bring their mother in.

So this is the "Catch-22." Any care facility, such as a board and care home, by law cannot give any medication to a patient without written authorization from the doctor. If you cannot go in to see the doctor, most health care providers will not issue the authorization – even for over-the-counter medication. The logical choice is to send someone out to evaluate her. However, this can only be done with the doctor's written authorization. The doctor will not give the authorization until he sees the patient. We were back to the beginning of the circle.

I was obviously getting nowhere with Mom's primary physician, as he refused to even speak with me. Every member of the health care provider staff that I spoke with expressed doubt that this was true, yet when I asked them to connect me with the doctor so I could speak directly to him, they weren't willing to do so.

I showed the social worker the empty prescriptions I was trying to renew from the hospice doctor we had seen when we had Mom briefly at the nursing home, and she suggested we try to get in touch with that doctor. The social worker called in her boss, who was the head of the department, and they both said they had no knowledge of any such doctor by that name.

After an hour and a half of them both mouthing the same platitudes that they "understood our problem and didn't want to seem unfeeling, but there was nothing they could do," they finally agreed to call someone further up the chain of command and see if *somehow* a Home Health Care practitioner could be sent out to evaluate Mom – the exact thing I had asked for when we had started.

As soon as I made it out of her office into the waiting room, I broke down in sobs and my sister Genevieve tried to comfort me as we made our way out the door. The lady who was filling in and had helped me at the front desk was concerned that I had apparently received no help and was so distraught that I was sobbing as we exited.

It was a great comfort to have had my sister with me so she could experience this frustration first hand. When someone lives far away, it's hard to really know or completely understand the circumstances of how difficult the challenges are. We both complimented each other on our efforts and knew that we had done the very best we could to try and resolve the situation.

Friday morning, I received a call from the social worker saying she was working on the situation. Hours later, I received the good news that they were sending someone out to see Mom. That afternoon, I got a call from Mom's board and care home saying they received a call that someone would be there in ten minutes. I rushed over and much to my delight, our doctor from the nursing home was there!

She had examined Mom, and was writing out all the authorizations we had asked for – an okay for pain medication, a muscle relaxant for Mom's twitches – and she called in the prescriptions for us. Then she called and asked the medical provider to put Mom on Palliative Care (used when the patient has a deteriorating medical condition needing symptom management at home and is expected to live 12 months). Because there was a waiting list, the doctor even asked to put my mom on Home Health Care (a less intensive home care program) until an opening became available for Palliative Care.

She was surprised that our other doctor didn't remember Mom and said she remembered all of her patients. But, of course, she had seen Mom just 18 months ago (versus four years), and had met all three of Mom's daughters when Mom was at the nursing home where she dealt with our unusual situation, so this doctor remembered us.

She was willing and even happy to be of service to

Mom. She gave me a card where I could contact her with a voice mail and said that even though she had been working for three years out of her office, she was originally hired by another location, and that must have been why the social workers said they didn't know of her. I asked her how they found her, as I doubted that the social worker was really going to try to help us.

We concluded, much to our delight and surprise, that it must have been the lady who was filling in for the receptionist that day – someone who was not even supposed to be there. Miracles do happen. Be kind to everyone – they may be the key to receiving the help you need.

Chapter 25
Preparing for Transition

"Act as if what you do makes a difference.
It does."
– William James

Despite our most tender, loving care, the disease progresses.

Even when you've spent a long time in preparation for the inevitable passing on of your loved one (at this point, almost 18 years since Mom's diagnosis), there will still be lots of emotions.

It was best for me to think about the final resting place of my mom on days when I felt strong. I wanted to have all of the details in place so I knew what to do when the time came.

I knew my mom wanted to be cremated, as she belonged to the Los Angeles Funeral Society which, comparatively speaking, performs this service at a very inexpensive rate. They give a list of service providers and their rates and you choose one that is geographically and monetarily desirable. When the need arises, you call them and they handle all the details. There is also a National Cremation Society.

If you want a casket, ask your spouse or a friend if they'd be willing to "shop around" for you, as prices vary dramatically. Federal law requires that, when asked, prices must be provided over the phone. Many people are not aware, but if you have the viewing within a few days of passing, there is no need for expensive embalming.

My father was an honorably discharged veteran and his ashes reside at a veteran's cemetery. At the time we interred his ashes, we also made arrangements for my mother's ashes to be interred next to his. If your loved one is a veteran or the spouse of a veteran, be sure to consider a national veteran's cemetery, as they provide a gravesite, a government headstone inscribed with the veteran's and spouse's names, dates of birth and death, and perpetual care, all at no cost to the family. (You only need to pay for cremation or other funeral arrangements.) Our VA cemetery has a lovely chapel where you can hold a memorial service, again at no cost. (www.cem.va.gov)

Professionally arranged flowers can be quite costly, so florist arrangements can be supplemented with potted mums from the grocery store. They are fairly inexpensive, yet their bright, large blooms are cheerful and create a lovely ambiance for a fraction of the cost. Most large grocery stores have a floral section with a selection of inexpensive potted plants to choose from, usually with colored paper wrapped around the pot for a finished look. They also have lovely, inexpensive bouquets you can arrange in nice containers and they look every bit as good as the expensive arrangements from the florist.

You may personally know a musician who can play at your memorial service. Many have portable keyboards, or just someone who plays an acoustic guitar is nice. You may know a singer who is willing to sing a couple of your loved one's favorite songs.

If you're playing a photo montage or video that you've made about your loved one's life, you may have already put music to it. If you're computer savvy, you can scan photos of your loved one into the computer in chronological order and add both music and narration to this lasting tribute. You can make a DVD and give a copy to the other family members who would treasure it as a loving remembrance. When I showed the video I made for Mom's memorial to my cousin, he said he wasn't aware of many of my mother's accomplishments, and was happy to find out about them.

When Mom started to fail again, it was time once more to get approval for hospice care. Because a residential home only cares for six people at a time, it's important to know that the state of California allows only one hospice patient per board and care facility, although once in a great while the state grants a waiver to allow two people on hospice at the same time.

I didn't originally realize that hospice is not an actual physical place where they care for people. Instead, hospice sends support people out to where your parent is living. They provide numerous services which are extremely helpful to both your loved one and their family members. For example, they offer your loved one nursing care, comfort measures and pain management. They offer *you* support to help you cope both before and after your loved one passes on, as well as tell you the signs to look for when the end of life is near.

After almost 18 years from diagnosis, Mom finally entered what medical professionals call "the active stage of dying." It can be characterized by several signposts. Breathing occasionally has long pauses of not breathing, and then resumes. The eyes can be open and yet not seeing, as if the loved one is asleep, but her eyelids forgot to close. The body may seem to withdraw from the outside world, sleeping most of the time. Eventually she will refuse food and drink, at which time it's usually just a matter of days. Once I was aware

197

of these signs and noticed them in my mom, it was very clear to me that this time was dramatically different from the other times we had been told Mom was near death.

All of a sudden, it seemed, Mom once again developed Stage 4 bedsores. Usually these can be brought on by not turning the patient frequently enough or by not changing wet diapers promptly.

As a result, the new social worker assigned to our case exerted tremendous pressure on me to move Mom to a skilled nursing facility, where she felt Mom would receive better treatment. She insisted that this was the consensus of the entire medical team. When I said "No," she was brutally blunt, saying that she did not feel that the current staff where we were was competent to take care of Mom and that I had no other choice.

To shock me into compliance, when the social worker sent the nurse to the board and care home, she told her to make me watch her dress Mom's wounds, thereby driving her point home with incredible insensitivity. This is a grueling experience which I recommend you avoid. The result, however, made it obvious to me that 1) these bedsores were not going to heal and 2) Mom obviously needed stronger pain medication to cope with the severity of her wounds.

Keep in mind that the medical staff may not correctly assess the amount of pain your loved one is experiencing. You may be more in tune with your parent's needs, having spent so much time with her. When I pointed out that Mom was grimacing when she was being dressed or when her diapers were being changed, they grudgingly had the doctor write an order stating that I could give Mom over-the-counter Extra Strength Liquid Tylenol. When I was told Mom had Stage 4 bedsores, I immediately asked for something stronger, and they increased her medication to Vicodin.

It still seemed woefully inadequate to me.

This is one of those instances where I had to don my "warrior's armor" to be my mother's protector. First, I stated that I did not believe we were without choices. I was equally blunt, asking if I correctly understood the situation that 1) Mom's bedsores were *not* going to heal and 2) Mom's death was imminent. They agreed that both these statements were correct.

I then said that it didn't make any sense to move Mom to a nursing home at this point. What would be the point of having a nurse checking her vital signs? It would not change the outcome. Mom already had the best hospital bed and once more the best inflatable bedsore mattress. Now was the time to make Mom as comfortable as possible until the inevitable occurred.

Having her stay in a loving home environment (the board and care) close enough for me to visit daily seemed far better than a noisy, impersonal nursing home. After all, what would be the point of having a nurse put her through the grueling process of cleaning her wounds twice a day? What Mom needed now was peace and comfort.

When I made it absolutely clear that moving Mom to a nursing home was not an option, they relented. The nurse deduced that, rather than the result of negligent care, Mom's previous Stage 4 bedsores had probably healed from the outside in, leaving some bacteria which spread inside and finally erupted through the top layer of skin. This was why the severity developed so quickly.

Now they suddenly stopped fighting me and agreed that

since Mom would probably pass on in a couple of weeks, it was pointless to move her. However, I was upset that I couldn't seem to convince the nurse to get stronger medication for Mom. I needed help, and I found it in my friend Judy, who seemed extremely competent at handling these situations since she'd been through the hospice experience with both of her parents.

Judy came to meet the nurse with me as my advocate and firmly stated, "Mom needs morphine *now*."

Much to my surprise, the nurse agreed to ask the doctor to write the prescription. "How soon will it be available for Mom?" she asked, and the nurse replied the next day.

Judy, who was sounding and acting very much like a health care professional, said, "It is apparent that Mom needs morphine now. Please see if you can get it by later today, so she can get some relief sooner." To my further surprise, the nurse again agreed.

I found out that morphine does not need to be injected. It can be put into a syringe without a needle and placed into the mouth where it can be absorbed under the tongue and through the cheek tissues.

What a difference! The next day, the deeply etched lines of worry and pain were gone, and her face looked smooth and relaxed. She looked so peaceful.

Now that Mom was facing death for the last time, I was more experienced and I could tell that her situation was far more serious than before. This time, Mom's 200 pound body had shrunk to less than ninety pounds, and her body had become rigidly contracted into a fetal position.

When I called my sisters this time, they didn't believe Mom was dying, since they had gone through this expectancy before. My sisters felt they had already said their goodbyes and didn't see the point in coming to visit what they feared would be someone who would be unaware of their being there. I could understand their hesitancy, as we had been told before that Mom was going to pass on, and it had turned out to be a false alarm.

The next day I met with the doctor and thanked her for all her help. Since the painkiller had to be administered every two hours, and Mom wasn't always awake, the doctor prescribed a morphine patch. "The patches are regularly used for people who require the drug over extended periods of time and not large, immediate doses. They release their active ingredient in gradual steps." (May 18, 2009 - http://news.softpedia.com/news/Morphine-Patch-Is-Very-Addi ctive-111829.shtml)

Mom's patch would automatically dispense the narcotic for three full days, allowing us to not disturb Mom.

The doctor kindly asked if there was anything else she could do to help me. Although I was somewhat intimidated, I asked her to call my siblings so they could hear from a professional that Mom was expected to pass on in the next few days. I thought it might be easier for them to accept this truth from the physician rather than from me.

Still, they chose not to come. It was near Christmas, and they had their jobs and loved ones who depended on them. Besides, it's a difficult thing to sit with someone who is dying, and it's not something every person is willing or able to do.

I could understand their position. From my personal point of view, though, it would have been a great comfort to me and very healing for our relationship to join together once more in our love for our mother, giving each other care and support in saying goodbye. The one thing Mom would still have been able to do with her presence, I believe, would be to unify us in our grief and love for her.

Chapter 26
Miracles Happen

"There are two ways to live:
you can live as if nothing is a miracle;
you can live as if everything is a miracle."
– Albert Einstein

Now was the time for me to tune in to the many miracles manifesting before me. One week before Mom's passing, I was given the strong urge to go visit her, even though I was on my way out of town on business. I paid attention to my intuition and was richly rewarded, as this morning Mom had that wonderful rally that you hear so many experience near the end.

Instead of the sallow pallor of days past, her skin glowed, she definitely knew me, and even gave me an exquisite smile. My mother was absolutely radiant in her beauty and clarity. There wasn't a line on her face. Her sparkling bright blue eyes focused on me and she clearly understood everything I said (that she was the best mother in the world and her daughters all loved her).

I quickly called my sisters to tell them about her rally and asked them if they wanted to tell Mom they loved her once more. Even though they didn't really believe me, they agreed to talk to Mom. As I held the phone to her ear, it was clear that Mom recognized their voices, and smiled at hearing each one. What an incredible blessing it was, especially since the past three weeks Mom had been mostly sleeping, and rarely had her eyes open for longer than a few seconds at a time.

This wonderful connection to Mom was the miracle I had not even known I was waiting and hoping for - I now felt it was okay for Mom to go.

The next day Mom had once again slipped into the stupor of the past three weeks, but it was a comfort to sit by her and hold her hand and spend time quietly recounting all the best memories of our shared lives. I sang all of her favorite songs to her and relaxed, knowing she was no longer in pain.

The last time Mom was conscious, I came in and, as I always did, I kissed her forehead and played "Nosey-Nosey," rubbing my nose against hers, and was blessed with another miracle when she actually managed to pucker her lips so we could share one last kiss.

On the night it became clear that Mom, as the doctors phrased it, "entered into the active process of dying," my Reverend sent a beautiful woman who played the harp for us. She looked and sounded like an angel, calming and comforting both Mom and me with the heavenly sounds of the harp strings, to help Mom pass peacefully into the next realm. (There are also groups of hospice bedside singers, such as Threshold Choir, you can access via the Internet.)

I was lucky enough to have a friend I could call to come and sit with me, to listen to the stories of the life Mom and I had shared together, and to just sit and "be" with me when I was done with talking. We closed our eyes and envisioned beautiful angels sitting on fluffy clouds playing the heavenly harp music we heard, beckoning Mom to come join them.

It had been almost a whole week since Mom had stopped eating and drinking, but she was still hanging on. My sweet Reverend Molly, who spent much time at Mom's bedside with me, comforted me when I cried that I wanted my sisters there. She said, "Maybe this is not theirs to do. Maybe this is for you to do."

Finally Reverend Molly, who shared Mom's last evening with me, addressed Mom quite sternly and forcefully, loudly saying, "Ollie, what are you waiting for? The ones who love you are surrounding you now."

Mom heaved a big sigh and relaxed. It seemed to be what she needed to hear in order to let go.

I had asked Mom to let me know when she was going. I was given another miracle at home late that night when I briefly was aroused from sleep to hear her spirit say, "I'm leaving now."

I replied "Okay", slipping back into slumber, knowing she was no longer my responsibility, as God would be taking care of her now. It was no surprise to me when the residential home called the next morning to say Mom had passed.

Knowing that I had already done everything possible for Mom, I felt no need to see her body, so I let her remains be transported to the mortuary. A few days later, I met with them to make the final arrangements. Know that the government sometimes provides a small death benefit to help cover the cost of cremation or burial, if you need it. If not, they prefer to save the funds for those who are really in need.

I called my sisters and they felt the perfect time for Mom's memorial service would be on her birthday, after Christmas yet before New Year's. I arranged for the church and called Mom's friends who were still living and invited them. The Reverend and I chose some wonderful readings, such as one from Kahlil Gibran's book, *The Prophet*. My dear friend from choir agreed to sing solo the songs that Mom loved best, such as the Lord's Prayer, accompanied by our church pianist.

I ordered one magnificently gorgeous flower arrangement to place on the altar. From the Dollar Store I found a dozen absolutely lovely candles and glass holders, so we could have the evening service by candlelight, supplemented by a few soft lights. The local party store had perfect paper napkins and small plates for after the service, so people could congregate to share their memories of Mom while nibbling on hors d'oeuvres. The local grocery had a fresh fruit platter and a fresh vegetable platter with dip that were so much easier to serve than preparing food. Supplemented by some baked cookies and beverages, the food was simple, easy and perfectly adequate. This is the time to be kind to yourself and do what's easiest.

I took a favorite photo of Mom to the copy store and had an enlargement made to display at the memorial. At the service, we showed the video I had made of Mom's life on a large television screen, and everyone said they were pleased to find out all that Mom had accomplished during her lifetime. Much to my surprise, several people at the service had only known my Mom *after* she could no longer speak. They stood up and spoke about how well they communicated with her anyway, and what a radiant smile she always wore, and how blessed they felt when in her loving presence.

None of them knew the story of her career – that she was the person responsible for the program that returned all the Navy seamen from overseas at the end of World War II and later that she was responsible for obtaining funding and seeing projects through for our California State University Northridge

"CSUN" sculpture sign and new Three Dimensional Art building, where she was honored at the dedication.

The memorial service was an opportunity for all of us siblings to honor Mom and to come to closure over her death. It was also wonderful to know that so many people cared about Mom besides us. A memorial service is a nice way to help you move on to the next part of your life, releasing your role of caregiver, and allowing you to accept the freedom this transition involves.

After the memorial, you need to endure dividing up the small amount of remaining possessions. Keep in mind that no matter how prepared you think you are for this, there will always be some discord around who "gets" what. Don't think that because you devoted a large part of your life to your parent's care, your siblings will think you should keep the remembrances that you desire.

I have to admit that I lost my temper. It was very freeing to express my anger at last over everything that had happened between my sisters and me during this long journey. In the end, I found that in a short time after they had gone home, I was able to release my anger, frustration, and resentment and let it go…another miracle.

This is what enabled me to do that: I realized I was blessed by all the years of closeness and wonderful times of being with Mom. In comparison to my 18 years of memories, my siblings would have only Mom's possessions to remind them of her. Once I embraced that understanding, it made it easier to release any remaining ill feelings.

I was given one last miracle to savor, and I fully believed Mom engineered it. When we three sisters took Mom's ashes to Dad's burial site where they were to be interred, I remembered the day Mom and I had come alone together to do the same for Dad. I remembered our discussion of how she had asked Dad for a sign, to let her know that all was well with him now. She suggested maybe a skywriter plane could write us a huge message across the sky, although we didn't see one at the time. (Later on, however, he gave us a different unmistakable sign, so we were content).

As I was thinking about this at the cemetery, I looked up and, much to my surprise, between two tall palm trees there was indeed an airplane skywriting a giant letter "S" hundreds of feet tall. Genevieve said, "That must be Mommy, saying goodbye to Sherry." The plane wrote another giant letter, an "H." As those are both my initials, we were now absolutely sure this was an unmistakable sign from Mom.

Many people will tell you that what you experience are not miracles, but just synchronicity. Believe what you choose. I choose to accept that it was my loving mother reaching out to her loving daughters, to let us know that all was well.

She was no longer trapped inside an immobile body that no longer responded to her. No longer alone in the isolation of a damaged, non-functioning brain. No longer afraid, her thoughts tangled and confused, unable to grasp a word or idea. No longer frustrated with the inability to communicate a simple need or desire. No longer angry that her fate was to linger so many years with continually diminishing capabilities. No longer grieving for lost abilities, lost friends, lost possessions, lost thoughts, and lost time. No longer would pain lines crease her forehead or cause her mouth to grimace, finally now released from agony. No longer robbed of her memories and left bereft in a wasteland of emptiness. No longer would we be able to comfort one another in person, but will now make do with memories.

Although grateful the journey is finally over, it is bittersweet, remembering all that has been lost.

I feel honored to have been my mother's caregiver and am truly grateful for many memories of times shared that bring a smile to my heart. I wouldn't have wanted to miss Mom's eyes lighting up when she recognized me. Our fun trips to the park to watch the birds fly overhead and feed the ducks in the lake. Our Eskimo kisses. How we all laughed and accepted Mom when we played Pass the Piggies and, not remembering what to do, she stuffed them down her blouse. Marching along to Peter Cottontail, and Mom clapping in time to the music at church. Singing to her. And most of all, finding a deep loving connection without words.

So while I honor the difficult times, I remember the challenges were overcome, and can at long last lay down the burden, knowing I am no longer in charge of caring for my mother – God is.

I take courage in facing the next part of life without Mom, by honoring the miraculous wisdom of my favorite childhood author, Dr. Seuss, who said:

"Don't cry because it's over.
Smile because it happened."

Appendix 1

Legal Form Examples

CMA PUBLICATIONS 1(800) 882-1262 WWW.CMANET.ORG

EMERGENCY MEDICAL SERVICES
PREHOSPITAL DO NOT RESUSCITATE (DNR) FORM

An Advance Request to Limit the Scope of Emergency Medical Care

I, _____, request limited emergency care as herein described.
(print patient's name)

I understand DNR means that if my heart stops beating or if I stop breathing, no medical procedure to restart breathing or heart functioning will be instituted.

I understand this decision will **not** prevent me from obtaining other emergency medical care by prehospital emergency medical care personnel and/or medical care directed by a physician prior to my death.

I understand I may revoke this directive at any time by destroying this form and removing any "DNR" medallions.

I give permission for this information to be given to the prehospital emergency care personnel, doctors, nurses or other health personnel as necessary to implement this directive.

I hereby agree to the "Do Not Resuscitate" (DNR) order.

_____   _____
Patient/Legally Recognized Health Care Decisionmaker Signature   Date

_____
Legally Recognized Health Care Decisionmaker's Relationship to Patient

By signing this form, the legally recognized health care decisionmaker acknowledges that this request to forego resuscitative measures is consistent with the known desires of, and with the best interest of, the individual who is the subject of the form.

I affirm that this patient/legally recognized health care decisionmaker is making an informed decision and that this directive is the expressed wish of the patient/legally recognized health care decisionmaker. A copy of this form is in the patient's permanent medical record.

In the event of cardiac or respiratory arrest, no chest compressions, assisted ventilations, intubation, defibrillation, or cardiotonic medications are to be initiated.

_____   _____
Physician Signature   Date

_____   _____
Print Name   Telephone

THIS FORM WILL NOT BE ACCEPTED IF IT HAS BEEN AMENDED OR ALTERED IN ANY WAY

PREHOSPITAL DNR REQUEST FORM

White Copy: To be kept by patient
Yellow
Copy: To be kept in patient's permanent medical record
Pink Copy: If authorized DNR medallion desired, submit this form with Medic Alert enrollment form to: Medic Alert Foundation, Turlock, CA 95381

213

Sherry Lynn Harris

Physician Orders for Life-Sustaining Treatment (POLST)

First follow these orders, then contact physician. This is a Physician Order Sheet based on the person's current medical condition and wishes. Any section not completed implies full treatment for that section. A copy of the signed POLST form is legal and valid. POLST complements an Advance Directive and is not intended to replace that document. Everyone shall be treated with dignity and respect.

EMSA #111 B (Effective 4/1/2011)

Patient Last Name:	Date Form Prepared:
Patient First Name:	Patient Date of Birth:
Patient Middle Name:	Medical Record #: *(optional)*

A Check One	**CARDIOPULMONARY RESUSCITATION (CPR):** *If person has no pulse and is not breathing.* *When NOT in cardiopulmonary arrest, follow orders in Sections B and C.* ☐ **Attempt Resuscitation/CPR** (Selecting CPR in Section A **requires** selecting Full Treatment in Section B) ☐ **Do Not Attempt Resuscitation/DNR** (Allow Natural Death)

B Check One	**MEDICAL INTERVENTIONS:** *If person has pulse and/or is breathing.* ☐ **Comfort Measures Only** Relieve pain and suffering through the use of medication by any route, positioning, wound care and other measures. Use oxygen, suction and manual treatment of airway obstruction as needed for comfort. *Transfer to hospital only if comfort needs cannot be met in current location.* ☐ **Limited Additional Interventions** In addition to care described in Comfort Measures Only, use medical treatment, antibiotics, and IV fluids as indicated. Do not intubate. May use non-invasive positive airway pressure. Generally avoid intensive care. ☐ *Transfer to hospital only if comfort needs cannot be met in current location.* ☐ **Full Treatment** In addition to care described in Comfort Measures Only and Limited Additional Interventions, use intubation, advanced airway interventions, mechanical ventilation, and defibrillation/ cardioversion as indicated. *Transfer to hospital if indicated. Includes intensive care.* **Additional Orders:** _____

C Check One	**ARTIFICIALLY ADMINISTERED NUTRITION:** *Offer food by mouth if feasible and desired.* ☐ No artificial means of nutrition, including feeding tubes. Additional Orders:_____ ☐ Trial period of artificial nutrition, including feeding tubes. _____ ☐ Long-term artificial nutrition, including feeding tubes. _____

D	**INFORMATION AND SIGNATURES:**

Discussed with: ☐ Patient (Patient Has Capacity)   ☐ Legally Recognized Decisionmaker

☐ Advance Directive dated _____ available and reviewed → ☐ Advance Directive not available ☐ No Advance Directive	Health Care Agent if named in Advance Directive: Name: _____ Phone: _____

Signature of Physician
My signature below indicates to the best of my knowledge that these orders are consistent with the person's medical condition and preferences.

Print Physician Name:	Physician Phone Number:	Physician License Number:
Physician Signature: *(required)*		Date:

Signature of Patient or Legally Recognized Decisionmaker
By signing this form, the legally recognized decisionmaker acknowledges that this request regarding resuscitative measures is consistent with the known desires of, and with the best interest of, the individual who is the subject of the form.

Print Name:	Relationship: *(write self if patient)*
Signature: *(required)*	Date:
Address:	Daytime Phone Number: Evening Phone Number:

SEND FORM WITH PERSON WHENEVER TRANSFERRED OR DISCHARGED

HIPAA PERMITS DISCLOSURE OF POLST TO OTHER HEALTH CARE PROVIDERS AS NECESSARY

Patient Information

Name (last, first, middle):	Date of Birth:	Gender: M F

Health Care Provider Assisting with Form Preparation

Name:	Title:	Phone Number:

Additional Contact

Name:	Relationship to Patient:	Phone Number:

Directions for Health Care Provider

Completing POLST

- Completing a POLST form is voluntary. California law requires that a POLST form be followed by health care providers, and provides immunity to those who comply in good faith. In the hospital setting, a patient will be assessed by a physician who will issue appropriate orders
- POLST does not replace the Advance Directive. When available, review the Advance Directive and POLST form to ensure consistency, and update forms appropriately to resolve any conflicts.
- POLST must be completed by a health care provider based on patient preferences and medical indications.
- A legally recognized decisionmaker may include a court-appointed conservator or guardian, agent designated in an Advance Directive, orally designated surrogate, spouse, registered domestic partner, parent of a minor, closest available relative, or person whom the patient's physician believes best knows what is in the patient's best interest and will make decisions in accordance with the patient's expressed wishes and values to the extent known.
- POLST must be signed by a physician and the patient or decisionmaker to be valid. Verbal orders are acceptable with follow-up signature by physician in accordance with facility/community policy.
- Certain medical conditions or treatments may prohibit a person from residing in a residential care facility for the elderly.
- If a translated form is used with patient and decisionmaker, attach it to the signed English POLST form.
- Use of original form is strongly encouraged. Photocopies and FAXes of signed POLST forms are legal and valid. A copy should be retained in patient's medical record, on Ultra Pink paper when possible.

Using POLST

- Any incomplete section of POLST implies full treatment for that section.

Section A:

- If found pulseless and not breathing, no defibrillator (including automated external defibrillators) or chest compressions should be used on a person who has chosen "Do Not Attempt Resuscitation."

Section B:

- When comfort cannot be achieved in the current setting, the person, including someone with "Comfort Measures Only," should be transferred to a setting able to provide comfort (e.g., treatment of a hip fracture).
- Non-invasive positive airway pressure includes continuous positive airway pressure (CPAP), bi-level positive airway pressure (BiPAP), and bag valve mask (BVM) assisted respirations.
- IV antibiotics and hydration generally are not "Comfort Measures."
- Treatment of dehydration prolongs life. If person desires IV fluids, indicate "Limited Interventions" or "Full Treatment."
- Depending on local EMS protocol, "Additional Orders" written in Section B may not be implemented by EMS personnel.

Reviewing POLST

It is recommended that POLST be reviewed periodically. Review is recommended when:

- The person is transferred from one care setting or care level to another, or
- There is a substantial change in the person's health status, or
- The person's treatment preferences change.

Modifying and Voiding POLST

- A patient with capacity can, at any time, request alternative treatment.
- A patient with capacity can, at any time, revoke a POLST by any means that indicates intent to revoke. It is recommended that revocation be documented by drawing a line through Sections A through D, writing "VOID" in large letters, and signing and dating this line.
- A legally recognized decisionmaker may request to modify the orders, in collaboration with the physician, based on the known desires of the individual or, if unknown, the individual's best interests.

This form is approved by the California Emergency Medical Services Authority in cooperation with the statewide POLST Task Force. For more information or a copy of the form, visit **www.caPOLST.org**.

SEND FORM WITH PERSON WHENEVER TRANSFERRED OR DISCHARGED

Appendix 2

Uplifting Supportive Music

Musical Inspiration

"Singing is a means to cut through gloom
and to bring harmony to the body."
- Paul Hasselbeck

When we listen to music, oftentimes the refrains of the words can replay within our conscious and subconscious mind. Therefore, listen to music that uplifts and supports you.

These are the lyrics to songs which I personally like for their strengthening and inspiring messages, and can be found at the websites given or online at music sites such as iTunes and You Tube.

Have fun adapting the lyrics to your personal situation. For example, when listening to the song "I Am a Hero," think of your father with Alzheimer's as the "king" and you can affirm, along with the song, that you will "protect the king to the end." To boost your courage and fortitude, replace one of the heroes named with your own name (for yes, you are a hero.)

Mark Stanton Welch
Reprint permission by Mark Stanton Welch
www.musicforeverysoul.com

I Am a Hero
In this life shall come Moments of challenge
When the shapes and the forms Tumble down
When the ego will writhe with Resistance
As the darkness does dance All around
When the child will reach out For assistance
From a God who seems So far away
Though everything's blurred, A connection is heard
A spark is ignited, A memory stirs

From out of the ethers in silence
From within the heart's Ceaseless void
A rider comes over the mountains
Emblazoned in power and joy
And the fog opens up like the Red Sea
A sweet song sweeps over the land
With rider and horse fast approaching
I remember like a hero I can

Chorus:
Oh set me upon raging rivers
Hang me out over the ledge
Turn out the lights if you must, but I tell you
This warrior shall dance on the edge
Nothing shall keep me from center
Fear shall be my greatest friend
I'll rise from the ashes
Of the choices I've laid
And protect the king till the end
For I am a hero, again and again

So I call upon all of you heroes
Whose spirits and deeds fill our lives
Inanna, Amelia, and Rachel,
Ulysses and Martin and John
Jamie and Michael and Peter,
Alea and Nancy and Ann
You and me, Gandhi and Biko
Come gather and join as we stand

Chorus

To encourage strength, stability, and flexibility

Mark Stanton Welch
Reprint permission by Mark Stanton Welch
www.musicforeverysoul.com

Like a Tree
Chorus: Like a tree, a strong tree
Reaching down, down, down
Solid on the earth
Connected to the ground
Let the wild winds blow
Let the storms rage through
I will bend and flow
Rooted to the Truth
Yeah, yeah, Oh yeah

Roots going down
Immersing with the earth
Energy rise, I Am rebirthed
Life Force flow, fill me up
Here and now I sing

Chorus

Trunk so solidly flexible
Etched by life so beautiful
In a balance between
Heaven and earth
Here and now I sing

Chorus

Branches reaching toward the sun
Gentle kisses from the One
Power of earth feeding fingers and toes
Here and now I sing

Chorus

221

To encourage peace and forgiveness

Lyrics: **Diana Meisler**, Caregiver
Music: **John Clement**
www.johnclementmusic.info

Soften My Heart
Reprint permission by John Clement

Soften my heart, Spirit
Let it not judge
Let it not grow cold
and bitter with resentment
Oh soften my heart

Soften my heart, Spirit
Replace fear with peace
Replace impatience
with forgiveness
Oh soften my heart

Soften my heart, Spirit
Open wide the door to my soul
Loosen the ties
I have chosen to bind me
Oh soften my heart
Oh Spirit, soften my heart

To encourage your ability to flow with life,
let go of expectations and embrace ease

Daniel Nahmod
Reprint permission by Daniel Nahmod
www.Daniel Nahmod.com

Water
I've seen my share of struggle,
When I thought that I knew best
When I've sailed through a storm 'Stead of stopping to rest
And it always seems hardest when
I've made up my stubborn mind
Well I'm changing my ways this time

Chorus: I wanna be like water Coming down a mountain
Into shadowy canyons, Flowing from pool to stream
Wanna be like water, Head uphill no more
I am bound for the sea

Have you ever seen an eagle
Head straight into the wind
He doesn't pick a fight, Spreads his wings and just gives in
And in the end he always makes it home just fine
I guess he knows that every storm subsides

Chorus

I'll let nature take its course, No more thinking that I know
Where this river's meant to go

I have railed against the stars
For the cards that I've been dealt
For the lottery I've never won
For the heartache that I've felt
But it always seems when I let go
of expectation and regret
Life has plenty of surprises for me yet.

To encourage trust and strength

Karen Drucker,
Dan Roth and Faith Rivera

I Will Surrender

I will surrender to my greatest highest good.
I will release any fear that blocks my way.
For every step I take is taken in pure faith,
and I am <u>stronger</u> every moment every day.

My mind is willing and my heart is open wide.
I trust my instincts and let Spirit be my guide.
I vow to live a life that's real and true and free,
as I continue walking in this mystery.

I will surrender to my greatest highest good.
I will release any fear that blocks my way.
For every step I take is taken in pure faith,
and I am <u>grateful</u> every moment every day.

There may be walls, there may be roadblocks in my way,
but I can choose to take a higher path each day.
And now I know that what I thought was safe and sound,
was only habit and regret that held me down.

I will surrender to my greatest highest good.
I will release any fear that blocks my way.
For every step I take is taken in pure faith,
and I am <u>kinder</u> every moment every day.

To encourage letting go, and embracing the moment

Faith Rivera
Faith supports caregivers with a free monthly concert at
www.faithrivera.com

The Power of Now
Reprint permission by Faith Rivera
© Lil' Girl Creations

The power of now is always present
Nowhere to be than where you are
The power of now flows oh so gracefully
The power of now is always perfect
Nothing to be than who you are
The power of now flows oh so easily

Be willing to let go
of everything you think you need to know
Be strong enough to let go
of everything you think you need to control
For everything goes away
Let everything wash away
The power of now…

The power of now is ever flowing
Connecting us all to the One
The power of now
unfolds so peacefully

Be willing to let go
of everything you think you need to know
Be strong enough to let go
of everything you think you need to control
For everything goes away
Let everything wash away
The power of now…

To encourage optimism

Robert D. Anderson
www.devotionsings.com

My Heart
Reprint permission by Robert D. Anderson
© Totally Intact Tunes, ASCAP

My heart is the start of love –
My heart is the start of love
When life all around,
feels like it's fallin' down,
My heart is the start of love

My heart is a home for joy –
My heart is a home for joy
When life all around,
feels like it's fallin' down,
My heart is a home for joy

Now I'm getting stronger, now I truly see
All I know for certain,
The change begins in me –
It begins in me

My heart is a place for peace –
My heart is a place for peace
When life all around,
feels like it's fallin' down
My heart is a place for peace

To encourage joy and peaceful acceptance

Robert D. Anderson
www.devotionsings.com

Maybe
Reprint permission by Robert D. Anderson
© Totally Intact Tunes, ASCAP

Maybe it's the sun shinin' through the rain
That somehow put a smile back on your face again
Or maybe it's the sea, breakin' on the shore
Revealing miracles you never saw before
Maybe these things changed to make you feel like you do
Or maybe it's inside of you

Maybe one small flower by a mountain stream
Suddenly woke you from a long unconscious dream
Or maybe it's the cry of a newborn son
That somehow healed a heart that had come all undone
Maybe these things changed to make you feel like you do
Or maybe it's inside of you

Maybe all this wonder, you think you don't deserve
But you can be assured that it's yours
Maybe all this started when you started to serve
And by giving, you only get more

Maybe a sad song with a tender line
Reached out & touched your weary soul & made it shine
Or maybe it's the love that you thought was gone
Returned to pick you up and carry you on and on

Maybe these things changed to make you feel like you do
Or maybe it's inside of you
Maybe these things finally changed,
the way you wished them to
Or maybe it's inside of you

Sherry Lynn Harris

*To encourage choosing love as your reality
and letting go of what others think*

Robert D. Anderson
www.devotionsings.com

What I Believe
Reprint permission by Robert D. Anderson
© Totally Intact Tunes, ASCAP

I used to think this world was just as it seems
I went crazy when I tried to change it
But after many years and miles, I've finally come to realize
I can simply change my mind to re-arrange it
And what I believe, what I believe
What I believe is true, is true for me
And what I believe, what I believe
What I believe is true may not be true for you

I've learned what seems to be, is not reality
'Cause whatever we desire we will see it
But we can get past this reflection to the mirror of the heart
Where our vision of this world is blessed by spirit
Illusion wears me down after awhile
Delusion would let me drown in denial
So if everything we see is only a dream
I must wake myself from this hallucination

'Cause when we come awake,
we understand only love remains
Then we bring this love to every situation
So what I believe, what I believe
What I believe is there is only love for me
And what I believe, what I believe
What I believe is true, is there's only love for you
And what I believe, what I believe
What I believe is true, is there's only love for me and you
Love for me and you

To encourage you to step up and do all you can

Robert D. Anderson
www.devotionsings.com

Do All You Can (Nkosi's Song)
Reprint permission by Robert D. Anderson
© Totally Intact Tunes, ASCAP

One little boy in Africa,
he put a face on AIDS
Told his story to the world 'til he died
And these are the words, the words he said

He said: "Do all you can with what you have
In the time you have, in the place you are
Do all you can - Do all you can"

Holy mother from India,
helpin' the sick and the poor
Somebody asked, "Why do you do these things?"
She said, "This is what I came here for"

She said: "Do all you can with what you have
In the time you have, in the place you are
Do all you can - Do all you can"

This is the gift they gave to us,
to share wherever we go
"Be the change you wish to see in the world"
Now I understand what they wanted us to know –

You can: "Do all you can with what you have
In the time you have, in the place you are
Do all you can - Do all you can"

Acknowledgements

"Sometimes our light goes out but is
blown into flame by another human being.
Each of us owes deepest thanks
to those who have rekindled this light."
- Albert Schweitzer

I am so grateful

To Molly Rockey and my Unity of the Oaks community,
for comforting me with ongoing inspiration
and spiritual fortitude.

To my mentor Andrea Gallagher who led the way
with loving compassion and professional guidance.

To Viki Kind for expert advice and encouragement.

To my coaches Grace Hollow, Alison Balter, and Bobbi Rudin
and healthcare professionals Dr. Alan Duben and Maureen
Hoeflinger, for supporting me through the process.

To Paula Cole, Editor extraordinaire,
for illumination and bringing cohesion to my story.

To Robert Pegg, friend for over four decades,
for computer wizardry and believing in this project and me.

To Elizabeth Godlewski,
my angel of mercy and compassion.

Index

About the Author

Sherry Lynn Harris is an inspirational speaker, author, and CD creator offering education, support and encouragement to Alzheimer caregivers.

Sherry had the pain and privilege of caring for her mother from the beginning diagnosis of Alzheimer's, through eighteen years, until her death. Harris learned by research and through trial and error many valuable lessons regarding how to take on the reverse role of parenting and caring for a parent.

She realized that her experience was not unique and that so many baby boomers are needing to adapt to the issue of the parent becoming the child. What Harris learned while caring for her mother was life changing and she felt it vital to share these discoveries "to inspire and lighten the load of others going through this challenging experience."

Additional support may be found in listening to the *"Serenity Visualizations"* CD Sherry created - located on the website www.Adapt2Alz.com - which can transport one from stress to peace in just a few minutes.

Sherry currently lives in Southern California with her husband Corey, and Harley, The Wonder Dog.

CPSIA information can be obtained at www.ICGtesting.com
Printed in the USA
LVOW10s1744280415

436425LV00002B/215/P

ML
7-15